The Music Therapy Studio

The Music Therapy Studio

Empowering the Soul's Truth

Rick Soshensky
Foreword by Jon Samson

ROWMAN & LITTLEFIELD
Lanham • Boulder • New York • London

Published by Rowman & Littlefield
An imprint of The Rowman & Littlefield Publishing Group, Inc.
4501 Forbes Boulevard, Suite 200, Lanham, Maryland 20706
www.rowman.com

6 Tinworth Street, London SE11 5AL, United Kingdom

British Library Cataloguing in Publication Information Available

Library of Congress Cataloging-in-Publication Data

Names: Soshensky, Rick, author.
Title: The music therapy studio : empowering the soul's truth / Rick Soshensky.
Description: Lanham : Rowman & Littlefield, 2021. | Includes bibliographical references and index. | Summary: "Rick Soshensky presents a groundbreaking introduction to music's power to heal and transform, weaving collections of uplifting case studies from music therapy practices with ideas from spiritual traditions, philosophies, psychological theorists, and music therapy theorists and researchers"—Provided by publisher.
Identifiers: LCCN 2021000128 (print) | LCCN 2021000129 (ebook) | ISBN 9781538154281 (cloth) | ISBN 9781538154298 (paperback) | ISBN 9781538154304 (epub)
Subjects: LCSH: Music therapy.
Classification: LCC ML3920 .S727 2021 (print) | LCC ML3920 (ebook) | DDC 615.8/5154—dc23
LC record available at https://lccn.loc.gov/2021000128
LC ebook record available at https://lccn.loc.gov/2021000129

∞™ The paper used in this publication meets the minimum requirements of American National Standard for Information Sciences—Permanence of Paper for Printed Library Materials, ANSI/NISO Z39.48-1992.

MUSIC THERAPY STUDIO

There is a place alive with creative energy for those
who seek healing, expression, growth, acceptance,
guidance, joy

There is a place to discover one's humanity, one's
worth, one's divinity
Where one may be honored
within a spirit of community, tolerance,
diversity, and respect.

There is a place for people who have been limited
Through all sorts of challenging circumstances.
People struggling with disabilities
People struggling with illness, personal
problems, social problems, trauma, poverty

This is a place for leaders
Who want to raise the vibration and light
Reduce fear, greed, judgment, competition,
and hatred
And birth more Heaven
In themselves and in the world

In this place we are not scared, intimidated, or
less than anyone

Neither are we better than or more than anyone
For we are all beloved children of God

—*Rick Soshensky*

Contents

Acknowledgments

I'd like to thank the following people for their help in making this book a reality:

Jon Samson, former student intern, now a Grammy-winning composer of children's music and successful music therapist, for his proofreading, editorial suggestions, and enthusiastic encouragement and appreciation for my work.

Ellen Levy, my cousin, and literary scholar, for her detailed proofreading and feedback.

Dave, my uncle, a talented artist whose terrible struggle with mental illness first started me thinking about the vulnerability of the human condition. In spite of his tormented and devastated life, he saved a percentage of his monthly disability check for me for over forty years. When this became known upon his death, it provided start-up money for my first music therapy studio.

Emanuel and Dorothy, my parents, now deceased, for their love, belief, and support—emotionally, financially, and any other way necessary to sustain my life. When I decided to start my own music therapy studio, they had total confidence in me. My father referred to it as *ein breira,* a Jewish phrase meaning "no alternative."

George, my brother-in-law, whose selfless generosity and Renaissance Man skills have improved the quality and manageability of my life so that I could get off the bottom rung of Maslow's Pyramid.

Lise, my sister, whose unwavering support, appreciation for my work, editorial feedback, and assistance in more ways than I can ever say, made this book a reality. Lise is the embodiment of the expression, "Love is a verb." Without her devotion of time, energy, and guidance, only God knows where I'd be, let alone this book.

Foreword

Jon Samson

If we're fortunate in life, we encounter certain people who unlock a piece of our potential no one knew existed. A part of us is seen for the first time, yet we can't see the full scope of significance until years unfold. It's also not often we get the perfect opportunity to express our deepest gratitude to those who have helped shape who we've become, and so those pivotal people may never realize the power of their impact. I am writing this foreword because for me, Rick Soshensky is one of those people. But before I tell you about how I know Rick, I'd like to first convey this—there are jewels in this book that may unlock or affirm something in you that is driven to understand, grow, heal, and embrace the full spectrum of the human condition.

You don't need to be a music therapist—or even know what music therapy is—to benefit from reading this book, though the clinical applications for doctors and mental health practitioners are abundant. The only prerequisite for diving into this rabbit hole of healing is a curious mind and an open heart, but even if you feel closed, I encourage you to keep reading. Rick Soshensky has a rare ability to shine a light on some of the most feared and abandoned crevices of the human condition—so if you think that might leave you feeling depressed or overwhelmed, just turn to any page and feel firsthand Soshensky's infectious sense of hope, humility, and passion for empowering others through music and authenticity. By engaging with these stories, you're invited to leave the confines of your own perspective and step into the shoes of a music therapist who has dedicated his life to working with some of the most challenging and heart-wrenching cases imaginable; to facilitate connection, expression, growth, and transformation when others thought it impossible or a lost cause. Rick's work and philosophy demonstrate what's possible when we hold another person's value—patient or not—as equal to our own; and as you begin to see things through this lens, you may emerge with an enhanced sense of compassion, exhilaration, and optimism for humanity. I know this first-hand, because Rick Soshensky was my clinical supervisor.

When I entered the NYU Music Therapy graduate program in 2003, I was an odd blend of anxious and arrogant, surely not ready to take on the responsibility of supporting others as a mental health professional. It would be one thing if the curriculum consisted of simply reading papers and doing research, but within a few weeks of my first semester, I found myself in a fieldwork placement facing children struggling with a plethora of challenges both physical and neurological. This is where I first met Rick. I observed him engaging joyfully—bringing out smiles, melody, and movement from children who might otherwise be sitting idle in a wheelchair or planted in front of a television. Rick modeled beautifully the brilliance of music therapy, but instead of being inspired, I left that day feeling unworthy. Truth be told, I was so internally preoccupied with my own struggles that I thought of forgetting the whole thing. I put in a request to defer for a year so that I could work on myself. But fortunately, some intuition beyond my insecurity was smart enough to realize that if left to my own devices, I would have just spun my wheels. Suddenly, staying in the program seemed like my best chance of working through my stuff, but that insight alone does not a therapist make.

As students advance in the NYU Music Therapy program, the therapists-in-training undergo intensive supervision while facilitating individual and group sessions. Shortly after beginning my independent work in the inpatient psychiatric unit of a New York City hospital, an administrator informed Rick they wanted me out. I was dejected. To be fair, it wasn't because of my work with the patients—we got along very well—I was more like them than I was like the mental health professionals, and I treated them like people instead of patients, just like I saw Rick doing—but due to my eccentricities, the administration simply didn't see me as professional material. At this point, NYU had serious doubts about me, but at a time when I felt most fearful that my self-doubt would be affirmed, Rick saw things differently. He believed my challenges were opportunities to deepen my learning process. He believed in me.

Rick opened up about his own healing journey and the integral part his pursuit and development in music therapy played in his own growth. To be clear, Rick is not someone to wallow in his prior wounds. He consciously chose to be transparent about his difficulties to give me hope and so that I wouldn't feel alone.

We'd talk at length about the Wounded Healer Archetype—the endurance and wisdom our challenges inadvertently create; how knowing what it's like to traverse our own suffering only hones a therapist's ability to empathize and recognize potential in people who are the most underestimated. Our conversations were inspiring yet grounding, and the quality of my work began to strengthen. Rick taught me how to view myself in the same way I needed to view my clients—with unconditional acceptance. However, we'd also discuss the fine line between embracing oneself and simply ignoring what could be improved.

No topic, no aspect of ourselves was off limits. This was so healing for me as I'd never encountered an authority figure who related with such authenticity. As a child growing up in Johannesburg, South Africa, I recall being deeply afraid of my teachers (except for my piano and choir teachers, go figure). While Rick was clearly the seasoned teacher and therapist in the room, he was always supportive, never patronizing. We both had an equal thirst for transpersonal psychology, healing, metaphysics, and mysticism. In my off hours, I couldn't get enough of audio programs by author and teacher Caroline Myss, so I'd bring her CDs into our supervision and we'd listen together and discuss how her teachings about consciousness could be integrated with music therapy. Our existential talks explored the parallel process of personal growth with clinical efficacy. We'd review the musical recordings I made with the patients, and Rick helped me put it all into context.

Toward the end of my internship, we listened to a final session I conducted with a six-year-old boy who had endured extensive trauma—but who also had an astounding ability to improvise songs that expressed his life experience, emotional landscape, and flights of imagination. His singing and storytelling was so powerful I had to hold back tears while it was happening. This patient and I had a musical dialogue about his dying mother and our own termination process. The child expressed his feelings about not wanting me to leave, but by the end of the improv, he expressed a sense of acceptance and resolution. When the recording ended, Rick said something I'll never forget—"That was perfect music therapy." Now obviously, that wasn't to be taken literally, but Rick trusted I knew how to interpret his words. That was his way of saying I had successfully learned how to not only put my baggage aside, but also use my talent to hold space for a person to feel, explore, express, and heal. I was now ready. This catalyzed my journey of recording improvised songs with children, which ultimately led me to open my private practice in 2005, CoCreative Music.

Even now, more than fifteen years later, I'm still unwrapping the gifts Rick has given to me. To this day, whenever I teach a workshop or speak with anyone interested in music therapy, I always ask: "What's the opposite of DEPRESSION?" Naturally, common answers are happy, joyful, and so forth, but the answer is, EXPRESSION! That was actually the first gem I ever learned from Rick, and it seems fitting to now leave you with that to ponder. The truth is, none of us may ever know the full extent to which we impact and influence one another. So it's my hope you not only derive meaning, positivity, and inspiration from this book, but that you'll share it with others.

Preface

Can anyone explain in mere prose the wonder of one note following or coinciding with another so that we feel that it's exactly how those notes had to be? Of course not. No matter what rationalists we may profess to be, we are stopped cold at the border of this mystic area. It is not too much to say mystic or even magic: no art lover can be an agnostic when the chips are down. If you love music, you are a believer.

—Leonard Bernstein (2004, p. 11)

Every once in a while, a TV reality talent show or news magazine show will feature an amazing musician with a formidable neurological, developmental, psychiatric, or physical disability; perhaps multiple disabilities. The members of the show and the audience are filled with awe as this person sings or plays an instrument with extraordinary ability, delivering a moving performance that seems miraculous in the context of the person's obvious challenges. The show is flooded with emails, texts, and calls. Social media and the talk shows are abuzz about this phenomenon for a while.

Here is someone who, in most other situations, might be counted out, might never accomplish the things by which most people define their lives. Would this person go to college, have a decent paying job, drive a car, get married, cook a meal, be a parent, stroll unaccompanied through the woods on a beautiful day, or even cross the street by himself? Maybe—but also, maybe not. Depending on the nature and severity of the person's condition, he or she may not be in the typical flow of life at all—

deserving of care and kindness hopefully—but without much visibility or relevance in the busy lives of most people. Suddenly, an outsider whose fair shot in life has been obliterated has somehow found the way back in; back to being someone who has a voice, someone who can connect, someone who matters.

Through music, this person has offered a little opening; a view beyond the mundane, a glimmer of hope in this cynical, scary world. We realize that magic is possible. That which on the surface appears to be broken actually carries the greatest gift of all. The spirit is undimmed. That Divine spark that is in everyone, creative, longing to communicate, to express, to connect, to experience joy, to grow, to contribute—it is always there and nothing can take it away. That is what is so inspiring. That's the message. People need this. We need to believe.

This is a book for believers, meaning people who believe, or would like to believe, that there is a door that opens to a world much bigger and more extraordinary than the one in which most people live. Maybe there are other ways to approach this door and walk through it, but we'll be looking at the way music does that.

I have been a music therapist for thirty years. I have a lot of stories, and I'd like to tell you a few. What do I do? I help people—primarily people with significant disabilities or those who have been through terrible trauma—to discover and express the music inside them. It's different for everyone, and there are myriad ways to do it. This thing that the general public sees now and then on TV—I see it, in ways large and small, almost every day. I seek communication with my clients' spirit. I am not interested in the broken, oppressed aspects of their personae that they, and everyone around them, knows only too well. I've witnessed, time after time, music's ability to draw in, uplift, empower, and reach those who might otherwise be marginalized, labeled, isolated, unreachable, lost. Music is a connector to the shining reality of their being that is far more boundless than they realize: *The Luminous Numinous.*

> *People are just as wonderful as sunsets if you let them be. When I look at a sunset, I don't find myself saying, "Soften the orange a bit on the right hand corner." I don't try to control a sunset. I watch with awe as it unfolds. (Carl Rogers, 1995)*

Music is much more than entertainment, a momentary diversion; it is more than the pop charts, one's favorite recording or musical artist or trip to a nightclub or a concert. Music is greater than the greats: greater than Beethoven, Bach, Mozart, Coltrane, Segovia, Hendrix. It is greater than they because the music moved through them just as we breathe the air, but we didn't make the air. Just as a ship sails through the waves but it is not the sea. Just as you move through your life but you did not create life. Music is like the air, the sea, life. Musicians are music's messengers but music is . . . well, what is it? That's the big question we will be exploring, but as Leonard Bernstein says: It's a mystical area or even magic. There is some kind of enormous passion contained within music; some kind of higher consciousness that is unknowable. We will have to be satisfied with that. That's what makes us believers.

When we hit on the right music, the transformative power it can unleash can seem momentous and inspiring, or it can be relatively subtle. Either way, there is a release from ingrained, habitual pathological patterns. We can write about these phenomena and come up with theoretical models to describe them, but ultimately, one can only stand back in awe at the healing and growth potential that has been released. Pioneering music therapy great, Clive Robbins (from whom we will hear much more), poetically called it, "The health and healing latent in the livingness of creative musicing" (2005, p. 12).

However, we can't simply say it's all just an unfathomable mystery and leave it at that. "The game is afoot," as my favorite fictional detective, Sherlock Holmes, would say. Like him, we will take out our magnifying glass and review the evidence—that is, whatever evidence I've been able to deduce. I've organized this book into three main sections that elucidate the inner workings of what I call the Music Therapy Studio. Part I, Music Therapy Studio: The Foundation, sets the theoretical groundwork for the principles to come as well as offering a little backstory as to how all this came into my life. Part II, Music Therapy Studio: The Framework, identifies the different components of music and looks at the through-line between conventional musicianship and music therapy. Part III, Music Therapy Studio: The Philosophy, examines some underlying principles and assumptions including esoteric and metaphysical concepts that explore the convergence of music and therapy, science and mysticism. At every step of the way, I will share a real-life story or two that illustrates how someone's life was transformed through a particular way of being in music.

What is a Music Therapy Studio? It is a space, permission, and whatever support people need to express and share themselves musically. It is a place for healing and the belief that the act of being in music and being creative is, by its nature, therapy. We, the practitioners, nurture and guide the process, but it's music that does the work. My development in the field of music therapy would ultimately lead me to the concept represented by the Studio as congruent with my belief that the paramount active principle in music therapy is, in fact, music. When I started my own business, I considered, but rejected, identifying the place where clients would come to engage in music therapy as a "Center," "Program,"

"Clinic," or "Service." I thought those designations could apply as easily, or more so, to physical therapists, MDs, social workers, or psychologists. The "Studio" is where musicians do their work.

However, if we are to call ourselves as music therapists, we are not simply talking about having a good time or improving at music. We are seeking to assess and address the core issues of a client's difficulties with the intention to help them achieve some functional improvement and personal growth. It is the music therapist's job to chart the right course. My experience has led me to a deep trust in music's power to transcend perceived boundaries and limitations.

At my first clinical placement, my music therapy internship at a psychiatric day program at a large New York City hospital, Paul became my first real client. He was in his late twenties and diagnosed with undifferentiated schizophrenia with autistic traits. He wandered slowly through the corridors of the program, attended his assigned therapy groups, didn't socialize, and didn't say anything unless directly addressed, and then, only a word or two. He was a loner on the periphery of the program, and people, both staff and clients, pretty much just let him be. It was known he had some musical inclinations, so we were introduced. When Paul and I played for the first time, I could tell he had talent. It's true that music is a language that is more fluent for some than others. In Howard Gardner's theory of multiple intelligences (1983), music is identified as an area in which a person might be particularly strong. Some people simply understand rhythm, melodic structure, harmonies, and musical styles. They don't need to be taught this. They just pick it up as people pick up their native tongue. It's natural for them.

Music was Paul's natural language, but nobody really paid enough attention to him to communicate or connect with him. On the occasional opportunity he did have to share his ability, he couldn't quite organize his musical intelligence in a form to which others could relate. As an example, I was told that the year before I got there, Paul had played an interminable "Jingle Bells Jam" on a little electric keyboard at the program's traditional Christmas talent show. Maybe for the first few minutes, people thought he was pretty good, but as Paul continued on, oblivious to his "audience," five minutes became ten. There was no indication that he was ever going to bring his piece to a conclusion, and someone finally had to tell him to stop. This year, as the Christmas talent show approached, the staff was making jokes behind closed doors about the prospect of a repeat performance. His ability was overshadowed by his disability, even to the clinical team.

Paul could use support, clearly, but we want to enter that mystic, magical place, if we can. I found a song Paul knew, not "Jingle Bells." It turned out to be the early sixties surf-rock instrumental "Pipeline." Paul could play the lead melody line on guitar as well as improvise around it. I played the rhythm guitar part, and we worked out an arrangement; a beginning, middle, and end. That was really the main help he needed to communicate musically. The talent show came and Paul was a major hit, getting an enthusiastic, sustained ovation.

He went on from there with my support—participating in individual music sessions plus every music group, writing songs, doing a couple other performances. And as his musical life grew, his visibility, participation, socialization, inclusion, and respect in his program also grew. I'll never forget the day I saw Paul playing pool with some clients and staff from the program. For him, that was a revelation! Then came the day that my internship was over. Paul raised his hand to share in the program's daily community check-in meeting (something he never would have done before our course of music therapy). In an angst-tinged voice, he announced, "Today is Rick's last day!" That is a painful moment every music therapist must face—one moves on to another job, another location, ostensibly abandoning this person for whom you have become a lifeline. But for that period of time, we had our amazing journey that will live forever in the annals of spirit.

In this book, you will read about numerous such amazing musical journeys. Music is a different realm of experience from our everyday, cognitively based awareness, and as such, it can lead to outcomes that wouldn't ordinarily occur and that can sometimes seem miraculous, as will be illustrated in some upcoming examples:

- A nonverbal and virtually mute client singing for the first time (Thomas)
- A profoundly disoriented and isolated brain injury patient writing a stunning song that others can share (James)
- A group of adolescents with disabilities giving an astonishingly confident and deeply moving concert performance, transcending their own and their parents' fears and insecurities (The Children's Performance Group)

What is the Music Therapy Studio to me? When you boil it down to its essence, all I really know are two things:

- Try to find the right kind of music and the right musical experience at the right time for anyone who shows up.
- The right music will take us to a better place than where we are right now (this is what makes me a believer).

As Leonard Bernstein poses at the top of this preface, "Can anyone explain in mere prose the wonder of one note following or coinciding with another?" Unfortunately, no. This is a book—mere prose. In any case, Bernstein says, if we try to explain music: "We are stopped cold at the border of this mystic area. It is not too much to say mystic or even *magic*." But I hope this book communicates some of that belief and some of that magic.

I

THE MUSIC THERAPY STUDIO: FOUNDATION

Introduction

Welcome to the Studio

ALAN: A SEARCH FOR COMPETENCE

I received a call from a case worker who said she had a client who liked music. A few days later, Alan walked into the Music Therapy Studio carrying a composition notebook filled with lyrics. He wrote songs, he said, played drums, and sang. Alan was forty-three years old and described himself as a person with autism. He lived independently in a supported apartment run by an agency that provided services for people with developmental disabilities in their local community.

As I became better acquainted with Alan over the next few months, I learned he had a drum set in his house growing up and had performed in some music shows while at a residential school for children and adolescents with special needs. He wrote a few songs as a young man while in a program to prepare him for independent living but didn't keep up with it. He picked up the practice again several years later during a long stint in the hospital while having a medication work-up. He continued writing after that and had completed quite a few songs by the time we met. He didn't have any way to go beyond the stage of writing the lyrics in a notebook and imagining the songs in his mind. He never thought he would have the opportunity to actually record them. So after some discussion at our first meeting, it became clear that was what we should do—make a recording of one of his songs.

Alan is the first case story in the book because his work in the Music Therapy Studio might be considered the most "studio" of all, in the sense that he used his sessions in a conventional manner—to write, rehearse, and record songs. We then make a music video and he releases the project publicly. An inquiry into what makes this therapy sets the stage for later examples and an understanding of music in all its forms as therapy. In our first few sessions, we established the basic pattern of working that would set the pattern for virtually every session after that. The whole process typically takes three to five one-hour sessions.

Step 1: Structure the Song and Make a Demo

Alan presented his song to me. He had the lyrics written down and a melody in his mind along with the style and feel of the music he wanted. The Southern Rock group the Outlaws was his favorite group, so everything we did had some connection to that. I helped him finalize his composition, figured out the chords to support the melody, and when he was satisfied with our basic arrangement, we recorded a demo with him singing and me on acoustic guitar.

Step 2: Record the Drum Track

Using my computer's multitrack recording program, we recorded a rhythm track with Alan playing the drum kit. Alan would sing while I played a rhythm guitar off-mic. The guitar and voice were minimally audible and were there to act as guides for later overdubs. The main task was to get a good drum track and a good feel.

Step 3: Add Vocal and Instrumental Overdubs

Alan recorded his lead vocal and I overdubbed guitar, and bass according to Alan's instructions. Then we both overdubbed additional parts such as background vocals and percussion. In future recordings, music therapy students would often help out with vocal or instrumental support.

Step 4: Mix the Recording

Finding the right volume balance for all the tracks.

Step 5: Film a Music Video

Alan wanted to make a music video, and we discussed ideas for it. This would include various shots of Alan singing, playing drums and acting a role in relation to the story line of the song, using the previously recorded and mixed song as the audio. In subsequent videos, sometimes additional acting and dialogue was filmed as a prologue to set up the song with Alan directing. Usually, I or, sometimes, music therapy students would appear as supporting players.

Step 6: Alan and I Edit the Video

Under Alan's direction we determined the right order of video scenes to compliment the song and synchronize any filmed singing and playing with the recording

Step 7: Release the Music Video

I published the video online and sent the link by email to Alan. He then sent it out to numerous friends, family, and professional support staff.

After four years of weekly sessions, Alan has completed three albums of twelve songs and music videos and is currently working on a fourth collection. We've uploaded his collections on a music sharing website, and he sends it to everyone he knows. He is a talented songwriter, and Alan's friends and family are amazed. But even though Alan likes to get accolades from people, I think it is simply making music that is most important to him; having this songwriter/recording artist as a part of his everyday life is very fulfilling. For Alan's family and social network, seeing him in this new light outside of his identity as a person with a disability was a revelation. One family member who wrote a letter to me commented, "The work you've done with Alan is astounding!" In considering what I actually did, yes, there was a degree of proficiency I learned during my years as a conventional musician. As a music therapist, though, my primary competence was in allowing and supporting what was already there in Alan to live and flourish. One day, as we talked about how astonished his friends and family were at his newfound identity, I said, "Maybe they thought you didn't have it in you." His response: "I did."

WHAT MAKES IT THERAPY?

I suppose most people can understand that such a process could be called therapeutic, but, in particular with music therapy, it is important to differentiate between the words *therapeutic* and *therapy*. A great concert or a campfire sing-along with friends might be therapeutic, meaning it would release stress, uplift one's mood, and create a short-term positive outlook. But soon enough, one's problematic mood or behavior patterns would return. Successful therapy would require something more long-lasting, where positive developments obtained in therapy sessions transfer to one's everyday life. I think we can see in Alan's story how music helped him to feel better about himself and gave him a framework in which to grow and develop. According to psychotherapist Michael Franz Basch (1988), the primary goals for therapy can be characterized as a *search for competence*, achieved through:

- Mobilizing and maintaining a self-respecting attitude.
- Furthering one's developmental process.
- Improving one's self-image.

CONNECTION, COMMUNICATION, EXPANSION

Alan comes to the studio to record his song in the same way and for the same reasons any musician comes to a studio, yet he always refers to his work with me as "music therapy," never simply music or recording or "coming to the studio." When I ask him what he means, he says it helps him express his feelings about issues that are concerning him. His songs have frequently confronted personal and social issues related to living with a disability, such as the loneliness of feeling different and people with disabilities facing prejudice in some way. Beyond this, as a songwriter, he has an awareness of his audience, and he is writing for them as well as for himself. He has verbalized this on occasion, saying something like, "I want to give people something new." Good songs also express important feelings for others.

Alan does not consider himself a spokesperson, role model, or advocate for people with disabilities. Although some autism advocacy ideologies would say they do not consider any neurological type to be superior or inferior to any other, Alan considers his autism to be a disability and says that if he could press a magic button and not be autistic, he would do so. He feels that autism impairs his ability to be more in the mainstream of life with better career and relationship opportunities. Although it is true that there may be discrimination involved in these barriers, through his music Alan has gained an expanded prominence in his social network. He showed me an email from another professional who works with him. It said:

Alan, your writing gets better and better each time you send it to me. Hearing your words accompanied by music is special. Please don't ever doubt your talent. I know Rick works with you to make this happen BUT this was YOUR vision. Please keep writing more. Make sure you send this to our Newsletter. People need to see and hear the great things you are doing.

UNCONDITIONAL ACCEPTANCE

Although I am interested in helping Alan make his music, as a therapist, I am interested in Alan's well-being and his personal growth. I maintain unconditional positive regard for him and his music. In addition to the introspection he gains from writing his songs, in the course of our in-studio relationship, Alan says things that many people might consider inappropriate; extreme statements of an antisocial, sexual, racist, politically incorrect nature. I think sometimes he is testing me to see my reaction as he often makes shocking statements with a smile. To a degree, it is dark humor, but still it reflects certain patterns of thought he has. Intrusive thoughts, he calls them. Most people would keep such thoughts to themselves. He blurts them out. He told me staff and other professional people around him would typically tend to censor him, saying something like, "Now Alan, you know we don't say things like that." I engage him at face value. I don't judge him, and I don't feel offended. He's never been hurtful to me or anyone else in the studio, such as students. As an artist myself, I like eccentricity and surreal conversation anyway. I have a relatively high tolerance for exploration of ideas, even outrageous ones, through language or artistic expression. We have fun. If he says something shocking or offensive, I might respond with my own humor, offer an alternative perspective, ask him a question or challenge his perspective. I'm offering him an opportunity to get his thoughts out in the open, to have some self-reflection, and to receive some feedback so he can consider and evaluate his ideas. I think he might be a little fuzzy on what one might call socially appropriate boundaries. Occasionally, I've felt the need to set a limit if I think his statements might be distressing or embarrassing to students in the room. He might ask "Why?" but he accepts it. If the banter becomes too tangential or unproductive, I simply say, "Let's get back to work."

COMMITMENT

Alan says he has a diagnosed anxiety disorder. If something in the recording process is not moving along perfectly (for example, he doesn't get something correct on the first take or there's a technical problem), he'll quickly become agitated, raise his voice, and say something like, "Oh no! We're never going to get this right!" As things like this come up constantly during the sessions, we've been through this scenario countless times. I reassure him that we've gotten through it before and we'll get through it this time.

He has improved in managing his feelings. Although he will often have an initial knee-jerk anxious reaction, he now composes himself very quickly, and we get back to work. The recording process takes time and involves inherent frustrations trying to get something the way you want it. On occasion we have had artistic disagreements or I have made technical mistakes. At times, I've brought up ideas or topics that Alan didn't like, and we needed to work it out. Through it all, he has always stuck with it.

This points to an important principle in the therapeutic alliance: commitment. When a client's anxiety, insecurity, or anger is triggered in some way, he or she may become extremely uncomfortable. The client has to make a decision whether or not to remain in therapy. Sometimes clients (or parents of clients) will make the decision to discontinue, with the mind-set that it's not working the way they hoped, or music therapy is not right for them, or I am not the right therapist. There needs to be a strong enough motivation to show up week after week, manage the anxiety, and carry on as one's comfort zone is continually challenged. Alan has demonstrated this again and again. He has worked hard and with dedication on all his projects. They are important to him.

GENERALIZATION

Successful therapy, according to psychotherapist A. Magaret (1950), is defined as leading to occurrences of generalization from the formal therapeutic session to outside, everyday situations, including:

- Changed Reaction-Sensitivities
- Increased Flexibility of Behavior
- Success in Handling New Interpersonal Problems

It would seem reasonable to conclude that Alan's experiences in the studio have had a positive impact on his ability to trust other people and situations and to manage his anxiety in other circumstances. His self-esteem and his esteem by others have been positively impacted. He has ongoing real-life experiences that have helped him to have greater insight into his feelings, thoughts, and behaviors. Alan is productive at a high-level endeavor, and his prolific output as a writer and musician continues to accelerate such that we have an ongoing backlog of two or three songs waiting to be recorded. His new work continues to improve and reflect his growth as a talented artist. There is an entirely new component to his personal and social persona. Noted mind-body psychotherapist Alexander Lowen (1975) defined happiness as the consciousness of growth. He believed that most people come to therapy because they feel their growth has been arrested in some way.

Alan has certainly made use of music therapy as a process of personal growth. I'm sure he understands this, although he may not fully be able to put it into words. When I asked him if he thinks our work in the studio has impacted his life beyond the music, he said, "I'm not sure. I've possibly gained some focus. I can stay with things longer." I think Alan underestimates his progress. Not long ago, I accidentally deleted a project from the computer that we'd worked on for several sessions and had almost finished. There was nothing to be done. It was gone. We'd have to start all over from scratch. Instead of becoming overwhelmingly anxious, accusatory, or despondent as he might have in the past, Alan accepted the setback, marshaled his resolve, and said, "Let's get to work." He made constructive suggestions; actually becoming more of a leader than any time in the past. With his proactive, positive attitude, we redid the project in two sessions, and it was an improvement on the one we lost. Now if that couldn't be called a well-realized search for competence, then I don't know what could be.

1

✣

My Journey into Music Therapy

WHAT IS THE RELATIONSHIP BETWEEN TYPICAL MUSICIANSHIP AND MUSIC THERAPY?

That is the question I've been exploring for my entire music therapy career, having started my life as a musician in a fairly typical manner as a singer-songwriter-guitarist. As a young aspiring professional musician, I spent countless hours "in the studio," working on my art: rehearsing, practicing, jamming, composing, recording. The studio might be thought of as a second home for a musician. In the contemporary terminology of disability awareness (most particularly in autism advocacy) there is a word, "neurotypical," that simply means not autistic or otherwise diagnosed with an intellectual or developmental difference. Although music therapists sometimes work with *typicals*, more frequently we work in psychiatric hospitals, rehabilitative facilities, medical hospitals, outpatient clinics, day care treatment centers, agencies serving persons with developmental disabilities, community mental health centers, drug and alcohol programs, senior centers, nursing homes, hospice programs, correctional facilities, halfway houses, and special education (American Music Therapy Association website). As such, the notion of the studio might be considered extraneous to a clinically oriented view of music therapy that places music in a secondary role, as simply a means to an end to achieve a clinical goal of some kind. But is it possible that something so fundamental to a musician's experience could be viewed as somehow superfluous to the music therapy experience?

However, in the term, music therapy, we must also acknowledge the second word—therapy—that, by definition, implies a rehabilitative, treatment-oriented approach to facilitate growth, healing, or improvement of some type. It may be difficult in our entertainment mega-industry, product-oriented culture to take music seriously as a treatment modality because it's, you know, music. Maybe some music therapists feel this way and want to be viewed as credible clinicians and, as such, de-emphasize music as a creative art, as they endeavor to apply music with precision, like a physical therapist recommending a specific exercise or a doctor prescribing a medication.

OH YEAH, MY SISTER HAS A RELAXING MUSIC APP: MISUNDERSTANDING MUSIC THERAPY

Just as practitioners within the field have contradicting views of music therapy, the general public may have even less of a clear grasp. Many people think music therapy is something you do *for* people as if music therapists are something like private performers to entertain, calm, or soothe their clients. Even people familiar with music therapy may have trouble conceiving it as therapy. While working at a music therapy program for children with disabilities, staffed entirely by credentialed music therapists, I consistently heard parents dropping off their kids saying things like: "Be good in music class and listen to the teacher." The staff held frequent educational workshops for the parents, but nothing we said could make much of an impact on this mind-set. Parents sometimes refer to my sessions as music lessons, even though they never heard me say that. Maybe they just want their children to go to a music class like any other child, and calling it music therapy is yet another painful reminder that their child is different.

On the other hand, there are music programs specifically for the special needs community that claim to enhance socialization, life skills, and development, and I've heard these programs referred to as music therapy, even though there is not a trained music therapist anywhere in sight. There are also arts for healing programs emphatically defining themselves as "not therapy" that are founded on the philosophical and political conviction that participants should not be pathologized. They should be empowered to take on active roles of expression and engagement to reinvent themselves as creative artists. From such a perspective, there might even be a contemptuous or competitive feeling toward people who obtained university training in music therapy.

Over the years, I've encountered all these versions and have had to come up with my working model, my truth. In some ways, I might not be all that different from the musician that entered New York University in 1992, except for the vast amount of contemplation and commitment I've devoted to my profession. I studied and received a master's degree and advanced post-master's training. I've been credentialed. I've researched. I've worked with countless clients and different types of people. I've written and published numerous articles. I've lectured all over the United States, as well as in Canada and Europe. I've taught at universities. I've mentored myriad music therapy students. That has to amount to something. There are so many influences that I integrated as I sought to join these two words—music and therapy—and all that entails. It is this area of inquiry that will inform our tour of the Music Therapy Studio. But first, let's go back, back, back . . .

BACKSTORY: SO YOU WANT TO BE A ROCK-AND-ROLL STAR

I came of age during the sixties and early seventies and was heavily influenced by the groundbreaking rock artists of that era—the Beatles, the Rolling Stones, the Who, Bob Dylan, Jimi Hendrix, and many others, as well as the folk and blues artists who preceded and influenced them—Woody Guthrie, Lead Belly, Robert Johnson, B. B. King, and Pete Seeger, to name a few. These artists made music that seemed to me to originate from a deep love of their musical tradition with a powerful impetus toward personal expression, artistic integrity, and connection with their audience that contained cultural and political implications. During the sixties and early seventies, the significance of music seen in this light became so extraordinarily important to me, along with millions of others around the world, that it amounted to a widespread cultural movement.

Music stood apart from other things I enjoyed as a boy, like being with my friends, playing sports, or watching TV. Listening to music seemed to be akin to a mystical experience, emanating not just from the radio or record player, but from somewhere beyond human reality. Sufi teacher and musician Hazrat Inayat Khan (1962) described music as a miniature of the harmony of the whole universe, for the harmony of the universe is life itself, and humans are a miniature of the universe. Of course, I didn't think about it in such sophisticated terms as a child, but looking back, even then I had this sense that music brought me into a higher realm. It felt like part of me, and yet, also connected me with something beyond myself; something powerful and profoundly alive. I listened as a focused activity with my full attention, rarely as something in the background.

I was drawn to the guitar. I don't know why; possibly because it was *the* musical symbol of the sixties, possibly for other reasons. In any case, there was really no question in my mind as to which instrument I wanted to play. My parents gave me my first guitar for my eleventh birthday, and I literally broke down and cried from overwhelming emotion, the only time in my life I have ever had such a reaction to a gift. It was as if I knew it would come to define my life. I started to teach myself, and I was highly motivated, practicing until my fingers bled, as the cliché goes, but true. I just had to learn how to play this thing. As I grew, I wrote songs with my friends and had the usual teenage groups. When high school came to an end, my parents encouraged me to go to college for music, but I demurred. I think it was just too personal for me or I was too insecure. I was having some emotional problems at the time and maybe didn't want to invite too much scrutiny or criticism. Nevertheless, I went to college and continued to play with friends and perform in informal and amateur situations. I pursued a psychology major, maybe because a beloved uncle had succumbed to hopeless schizophrenia, and I wanted to understand more about the recesses and vulnerabilities of the human mind. But, in general, college was just something to do, like a continuation of high school. My heart and focus weren't fully in it, as I unenthusiastically completed my undergraduate studies.

As I searched for something upon which I could base my emerging adult persona, music was the only thing that felt real to me. I had no choice, I decided. I had to become a professional musician. I moved into a cheap apartment in New York City and began working diligently on my music, taking multiple lessons, collaborating with other musicians, writing songs, putting in long hours of practice, and playing for an audience anywhere they would let me. My ambition quickly grew to be an "artist that mattered," like the ones that were so important to me growing up. My first idea was to be a rock singer/songwriter/guitarist behind a great group, like Pete Townshend of the Who. But then I thought I could be the front man myself, like Tom Petty or Bruce Springsteen. Or maybe even the whole genius, greatest-of-all-time like Jimi Hendrix or the biggest in the world like the Beatles. I sought immense stardom, but I shortly realized, playing out in New York City by myself and with groups, that just about everyone had the same idea. We were all "the next big thing."

For someone who stood out as a teenager and in college because of my musical talent, it was intimidating and overwhelming to be just one of thousands of aspiring superstars. But I was the real thing and most of them were not, I decided (just like we all did). So in spite of the seemingly insurmountable odds, I made recordings of my music, sent demos to music industry people, and hustled for gigs. Actually, gig, being musician slang for job, was something of a misnomer, since most clubs in Manhattan paid little or nothing for original artists, such was the preponderance of ambitious musicians. In fact, some of the rock clubs for original musicians in New York City at the time actually had a "pay to play" policy, requiring the musicians to pay the light person, sound person, and so on. This was eventually stopped by the musicians union.

In order to feel like a professional musician and also to avoid working as temporary office help or a waiter, I tried to get decent paying gigs, playing cover songs in bars and playing music for dancing at parties and weddings. As time went on, I started to make a reasonable living at this, eventually moving into the upper echelon of the club date business. I became a featured rock singer/guitarist in the top New York society dance bands, playing at numerous world-class social events of the rich and famous, including, to name a few of the more prominent "gigs," Malcolm Forbes's so-called Party of the Century at one of his mansions, the Royal Wedding of Prince Andrew and Sarah Ferguson, and Queen Elizabeth's Birthday Ball at Windsor Castle. This might sound glamorous, but, as many people who find themselves in seemingly enviable positions discover, what seems exciting from the outside is not always so great from the inside. Although I always liked playing music, the band leader was an extremely controlling, occasionally abusive, person, and the other musicians, like me, felt discontent and cynical using our talents to crank out recognizable hits for dancing, no matter how illustrious the gig.

Unfortunately, I wasn't doing so well on the original artist front. It is notoriously difficult to make an impact in New York City, of course. I found a little success—recordings of my music were occasionally played on college or noncommercial radio; I had a few fans in some out-of-town venues; but, in general, my songs, my presence, my playing didn't seem to be affecting audiences or standing out the way I believed they should or, at least, was hoping they would. In spite of a little industry interest from time to time, it all seemed to fizzle out, and I didn't seem to be able to muster the necessary confidence or relentlessness with the music business to break through. I began to fear a possible future professional life as a hack, an aging bar and wedding singer. But what else could I do?

PARADIGM SHIFT: MY DISCOVERY OF MUSIC THERAPY

My father knew I was searching, and one day he called me on the phone and said he had seen something about music therapy on TV. He said, "This is what you're looking for. I *know* this is for you." That was the way my father was. He didn't say, "You might want to look into this," or some other type of suggestion. He said he knew. I wasn't quite as convinced, but I did respect his judgment and intentions enough to look into it.

For some reason, I had never heard of music therapy. I didn't know it existed as a profession. I thought if it was viable for me, it would, at most, become an adjunct to my performing work. With my dream of becoming a successful original artist not yet materializing and feeling like just another wannabe in the clubs, I was always living for someday. "Someday my music will mean something to people"; "Someday I'll be somebody." I remember thinking that music therapy was my way out of "someday." I couldn't stand to wait for "someday" anymore. Playing dance music for tipsy partiers wasn't enough for me. I needed to make a more substantial contribution *right now.*

Although my desire to be a rock star had certain altruistic motivations, to give people joy and to create music that was emotionally meaningful, it also had some more worldly and self-centered incentives. Fame and fortune, of course; power to control others; attractiveness to women without having to risk rejection; nurturing and exposing my neurotic troubles through songwriting and being praised for it, rather than attempting to heal my emotional problems. A second thought I had was, "The music in music therapy is primarily for the healing benefit of others, not for the fulfillment of my own ego."

- The need to make a contribution right now
- The healing of others through music taking precedence over my own self-aggrandizement

It was these two thoughts combined that propelled everything forward and shifted the entire direction and focus of my life. It was, in fact, a personal paradigm shift—a transformation, a metamorphosis, a change from one way of thinking to another. William James (1901) said that by changing your mind, you can change your life and discussed the idea of a quantum shift in *The Varieties of Religious Experience*. James's work was also a primary source in the development of *Alcoholics Anonymous*, which holds, "There is only one key and it is called willingness" (12&12, Step Three, 34). *A Course in Miracles* (1975) suggests that the world is nothing in itself. Your mind must give it meaning. . . . Change your mind and all the world must change accordingly.

BACK TO SCHOOL: WELL, NOT SO FAST

I found out that New York University had a music therapy master's degree program. That's all I knew. I didn't really know what music therapy was or what music therapists did. I didn't know there were different schools of thought or different approaches in the field. I certainly didn't know about the new American Association for Music Therapy having split off from the original National Association for Music Therapy in 1975, based on ideological differences as spearheaded by New York University (they joined back together as one association, the American Music Therapy Association, in 1994). I didn't know about anything.

But as NYU was the only possibility I did know about, I decided to make an appointment to talk to somebody. When the faculty member I spoke with very kindly asked me which clinical population I might be interested in working with, I understood enough to think one thing—I had no interest in referring to anybody as a *clinical population*. So when we finished our meeting, I thanked her and walked out knowing this wasn't for me.

I was in my mid-30s at this point and starting to feel the pressure of time bearing down on me. I had played music in institutions for years: hospitals, psychiatric wards, homeless shelters, and nursing homes, occasionally as a volunteer but usually for pay. At the time, it might have been just another gig, another place to play, but I could tell I was good at it. I had an empathetic streak for people in rough situations, and I seemed to have a knack for helping them to feel comfortable and drawing them into the music. I saw how they became more alive, more healthy while in music. I loved that. The emotional pain of another year of unfulfilling bar and party work and not making any substantial headway on the original artist front caused me to reconsider my stance on the clinical population objection. I dipped my toe a little further into the music therapy pool and found a job playing in a nursing home twice a week.

WILLIAM: UNFORGETTABLE

I eventually crossed paths with William, an African American man in his 70s with advanced dementia. He was in a wheelchair and could not speak or take care of himself in any way. His face showed no expression, and every day the nurses would dress him, feed him, and wheel him into a corner of the dayroom where I would play. For the most part, he would stay there until they put him to bed. I never noticed him until one day, as I was singing the Nat King Cole song "Unforgettable," I heard a gruff, Satchmo-like voice coming from the corner of the room singing: "Unforgettable, that's what you are. . . ." It was William, and he was lit up with a grin that covered his whole face. I found he knew all the words and soon discovered he could sing many other songs as well. I always thought it was so paradoxical that a man with fading memory found a way to emerge by singing a song called, "Unforgettable." Here was a man in late-stage dementia who had lost all ability to communicate, required total assistance with all personal care, and was unable to function in any way. Yet he came alive in music and could sing a whole repertoire of songs. With feeling! The nurses wouldn't believe it until they saw it for themselves. They came from all over the facility to witness William singing, and he was glad to oblige. Following a music session, William was more animated and had increased ability to communicate.

William was not the only resident I met for whom music had this wondrous effect. I know now that this is a common phenomenon that music therapists experience every day, but at the time, it was a revelation. That sealed the deal for me. These early experiences made it clear to me that music was not simply entertainment; that, in fact, something far more powerful and profound was going on. I wanted to learn more. I wanted to do this.

CLINICIAN: WHO, ME?

I took the audition at New York University, and next thing I knew, I was sitting in my first class. I began to hear this word—clinician—used with great frequency. I wasn't sure I liked that word, at least as applied to me, and struggled with what it meant. I knew I could provide people with access to enjoyable musical experiences, but was I a clinician? What was music "therapy"? I pondered these questions. Certainly, my love of music and ability to play it had enriched me, given me direction, and been an indispensably essential aspect of my life. But as any musician knows, there's music, and then there's the rest of your life. One doesn't need to look too far to find even successful musicians whose musical experiences could not save them from a descent into addiction, psychological problems, failed relationships, and other pitfalls of life that brought them into the abyss of despair and even death. Not to mention the countless others—and I could have been one of them—whose love of music but failure to find adequate success or appreciation obliged them to deal with poverty and feelings of failure. No, it seemed music, in and of itself, was not a panacea. Or maybe music was pure and healing, but it was the music "business" that was the problem. Or maybe, as M. Scott Peck (1978) says in the first line in his famous book, *The Road Less Traveled*, "Life is difficult." That's it and there's no way out.

LIFE IS DUKKHA

Life will break you. Nobody can protect you from that, and living alone won't either, for solitude will also break you with its yearning. You have to love. You have to feel. It is the reason you are here on earth. You are here to risk your heart. You are here to be swallowed up. And when it happens that you are broken, or betrayed, or left, or hurt, or death brushes near, let yourself sit by an apple tree and listen to the apples falling all around you in heaps, wasting their sweetness. Tell yourself you tasted as many as you could.

—Louise Erdrich (2005)

We strive, we hope, we love, we lose, we suffer, we cry. Sometimes we give up. Ultimately, as the Buddha taught in the first Noble Truth, "Life is Dukkha," which is often misunderstood to mean life is suffering, but actually more closely means that life is incapable of satisfying. We identify with things that are ephemeral and insubstantial: our bodies, our opinions, our habits, our feelings, our sense perceptions, our relationships, our struggles, our successes. Dukkha colors everything. Even behind good feelings, lucky breaks, and happy times, there is this nagging, underlying angst: it won't last. And, of course, we know that no matter what, we are powerless before our impending death.

Amazingly, when we make music out of our pain, we find our power. We can manage. African American songs developed in the era of slavery were sung to remind the Africans of home or as a means of withstanding hardship or expressing anger through creativity or covert opposition. Beethoven revealed that in response to the despair of his increasing hearing loss, he would "seize fate by the throat; it shall not bend or crush me completely." He allegedly called the 5-5-5-minor 3rd, "Da-Da-Da-Dum" opening to his 5th Symphony—arguably, the most famous musical theme in Western music—the struggle with "Fate" when it "knocks at the door." "I'm So Lonesome, I Could Cry," sang Hank Williams. "All Things Must Pass," sang George Harrison. "Death Don't Have No Mercy," lamented Reverend Gary Davis. Why does this music endure when it arises from things we dread? For one thing, at least it gets things out in the open. These agonizing feelings are no longer our own private misery. We become connected, and that in itself is deeply comforting. But music is more than a channel for our collective suffering. Music is a transformer. It is the bridge between the physical and the spiritual.

Music is the language of the spirit. It opens the secret of life bringing peace, abolishing strife. —Kahlil Gibran (2009)

When we take the most difficult feelings of life and set them to music—sing them, play them, make chords, melodies, and rhythms that reflect them—then we know, in the deepest, most real and enduring part of us, that these things that torment us are, in fact, not really true. We have mastery over them. They cannot overwhelm us. They are not bigger than us.

Even death. It is the reverse of Dukkha. Although we face pain and hardship, just beyond, there is beauty. It says in *A Course in Miracles* (1975):

> *Nothing real can be threatened.*
> *Nothing unreal exists.*
> *Herein lies the peace of God.*

I believe through music, we touch this truth. I felt there had to be a way to utilize music in all its fullness as a profound human experience to help people deal with the dreadful struggles of life. And thus began my journey into the field of music therapy.

2

Music Therapy Studio

The term studio, as it applies to the creative arts, typically refers to a workspace utilized for instruction, rehearsal, experimentation, preparation, and development, such as an art studio, recording studio, rehearsal studio, film studio. It might be considered a private place, restricted to essential personnel, where creative work is conducted prior to its readiness for public presentation. In the professional music world, a major recording studio might be a highly stressful and competitive environment, due to the excessive degree of money, ego, and career aspirations on the line. In its more idealistic form, however, a studio can be considered a safe, nonjudgmental place for the creative process to unfold. Ideas can be tried, reworked, scrapped, and redone until something satisfying takes form. A music studio would be a place to engage in the activities intrinsically associated with a musician's experience. Perhaps there may be other classifications of musical activity, but they could probably be included as subcategories of the following.

ACTIVITIES OF MUSICIANS

Instruction—Usually one teacher for one or more students, with the purpose of improving technical competencies of the student(s).

Rehearsal/Practice—An activity to improve technical facility. Repetitive exercises for the purpose of mastery of skills, physical dexterity, motor control, speed, familiarity with scales and intervals, tone, accuracy of pitch, and so forth. Or one or more players with the goal of mastering a specific full piece, for the purpose of personal improvement or some form of public rendition.

Jamming—Musicians getting together to explore musical interaction, ideas, and communication through an improvisatory approach. Not specifically goal-oriented toward practice, composition, or rehearsal. Could take place in a studio or in a concert.

Composing—Can be solitary or collaborative. The goal is to reach into the realm of personal and collective musical expression to create a piece of emotional meaning for one's self and, it is hoped, others.

Recording—To capture an effectively rendered, moving performance of a piece of music. Previous to the advance in home recording technology, this was necessarily collaborative but now can also be a solo endeavor. Its implied purpose is generally for sharing with others.

Public forms of music are also part of the complete picture of musical activity. The following may take place in a studio (such as a concert recorded for radio or TV), but more typically they take place in larger public settings:

Performance—To share, communicate, entertain, and possibly impress. Generally, this involves a clear demarcation between performer and an audience that can range from several to hundreds of thousands. It can also include recorded or transmitted audio or video performance (such as radio, TV, or movies), in which case the potential audience may be well into the millions.

Ritual—Music for bringing people together or enhancing a certain concept or event, such as a wedding celebration, music for nationalistic or religious/spiritual purposes, or even a living room singalong among friends. It can have a divine quality, placing people in communication with forces beyond the human. In pre-industrial cultures, it may have been bound up with survival, such as a Harvest Ceremony or War Dance. Typically, it involves high levels of participation, with less separation between audience and performer than in a typical performance situation.

WHICH WAY DO WE GO?

That way is a very nice way. Of course, people do go both ways. That's the trouble. I can't make up my mind.

—*Scarecrow, from* The Wizard of Oz

With all these options, how does the practitioner know in which direction to go? Although experience, judgment, intuition, empathy, musicianship all combine to forge a path, the answer will reside in the client. They will let us know, if we are open, observing, listening, and flexible. This book will explore detailed examples of each approach and how it arose.

If the practitioner can be a watcher rather than a show-er, a seeker rather than a know-er, a listener rather than a teller, the way will present itself. The great spiritual teacher Krishnamurti (1992) reminds us:

We do not listen. There are too many noises about us; inside us, there is too much talk, too much questioning, too much demanding, too many urges, compulsions. We have so many things and we never listen to any one of them completely, totally, to the very end. And if you would kindly so listen, you will see that, in spite of yourself, the mutation, that emptiness, that transformation, the perception of what is true, comes into being. You don't have to do a thing, because what you do will interfere, because you are greedy, you are envious, you are full of hate, ambition, and all the mischief that thought can make. So if you can listen happily, effortlessly, then perhaps in the quiet, deep, silence you will know what is truth. And it is only that truth that liberates, and nothing else.

DIGGING THE WELL

While in the midst of my many musical relationships, I had no idea what wonderful developments, if any, would transpire. I devoted my attention, my compassion, my acceptance, my optimism, to the work. To be looking for it, to stay present—to try this, try that—to attempt to make music with a client who seems like it might be the right kind of music and approach for that client at that time—that is the essential skill. As the Buddha taught, according to prominent New Age author Deepak Chopra (2007):

When you dig a well, there's no sign of water until you reach it, only rocks and dirt to move out of the way. When you have removed enough; soon the pure water will flow. —*Buddha*

These moments of breakthrough when they show up may be characterized as a quantum shift, meaning an abrupt change, sudden increase, or dramatic advance, without seeming to move observably from one place to another. Like the creative act itself, something is there that was not there before—a different person with a different identity in the world. But one has to work for it, experiment, struggle, hang in there, have fun along the way.

It might seem as if nothing much is happening and then, suddenly, the client is not the same as he or she was moments before. He or she has moved out of the confines of pathological limitation, social perception, and labeling. The experience might have qualities in common with what the great humanistic psychologist Abraham Maslow (1968) called, "Peak Experiences"—a brief but intense increase in personal awareness, positive feeling, and capability that can serve as a turning point in a person's life. Whatever one calls them, they are not manufacturable. Our work in the studio lies in finding ways to prepare clients, to situate them so these moments have the potential to emerge.

This is not to make exaggerated claims that music therapy always results in sudden and dramatic transformation of serious conditions. The work takes time, occasionally a lot of time, as with Owen, a nonverbal sixteen-year-old boy with severe autism, who over a period of years, progressively became capable of enjoying himself in music, finding an important channel for relationship, self-acceptance, and self-expression. However, even with Owen, I could point to certain moments of sudden developmental shift. As an example, for years, he wouldn't even go near a full drum kit. If I suggested it or led him to it, he would withdraw. One day I tried it again, thinking probably like all the other times, he wouldn't accept. But I keep on digging the well. This time he sat down, and we jammed for twenty minutes, he on the drums, I on guitar. After that, we would do it often. There are reasons why that is important for him: being willing to take on an intimidating challenge, trusting in the relationship, accepting and not withdrawing, having a substantial rather than fleeting engagement, perhaps others.

THE FOUR EXPERIENTIAL STATES OF MUSIC THERAPY

You can expect to hear a lot about the pioneering music therapy team of Clive Robbins and Paul Nordoff in this book. Dr. Clive Robbins was my most inspiring teacher and mentor. Paul Nordoff passed away before I entered the field but through their collaborative writing, they became and remain my most important influences. Prominent music therapist and researcher Dr. Ken Aigen (1993) has discussed four distinct experiential states with which a practitioner can expect to contend, as categorized by Nordoff and Robbins. Although the following terms were somewhat informal-sounding, coming out of a classroom situation as they did, they are referred to as:

The "Real Thing"—That moment of transcendence where the therapist and client are living in the "creative now" together at the deepest level of the reality of music. It can be transformative, but cannot be predicted, forced, or sustained beyond the realization of the individual content that is achieved.

The "Next Best Thing"—Ongoing confidence and skill building; a significant level of musicality and possible entry point to the "real thing," but more of a "working experience." It provides insight, builds resources, and creates stability.

"Just Coping"—"Slogging Along"—Working to handle a difficult clinical situation in which the direction or outcome is not at all clear; there may be considerable tension and possibly boredom (but out of the very unpredictability of the situation, the "real thing" may be triggered and bring resolution).

"Confusion"—A possible volatile or demanding clinical challenge in which the therapist may be missing opportunities or just doesn't know what to do.

Of course, as music therapists, we would like the real thing all the time, but we will have to accept that it's not possible. In therapy situations characterized by confusion, just coping, or the next best thing, creative moments present themselves to the therapist who has his or her antennae out for an entry point into deeper levels of contact—a matched rhythm, an interesting melodic idea, a relationship dynamic or activity that suggests a song, a lyrical or stylistic idea introduced by the client, even a random intuition. It is essential that the therapist learns to recognize and take advantage of these moments; otherwise the clinical work can stagnate and become mired in just coping and confusion. Paul Nordoff (in Aigen, 1993) said:

The basic truths lie in music and lie in the ability of the human being to respond to it. And here we have on one side, music; here we have on the other, pathology and how the pathology is hindering the child's musical response. With music, we work to overcome this hindrance and bring the child into musical experience that will be meaningful and significant for him. (p. 16)

BEYOND ENTERTAINMENT

> *Felipe Herrara, a Chilean bank president, tells of a tiny Indian village he'd visited on a feasibility study for a proposed hydroelectric dam. Since the village lacked virtually every modern development, Herrara asked the local chiefs what project the bank could fund as a gift in gratitude for their hospitality and assistance. After some deliberation, the chiefs concluded, "We need new instruments." The astonished bank president replied, "Maybe you don't understand. We would like to help you with improvements like electricity, running water, sewers, telephones." But the chiefs had understood the offer. "In our village," it was explained, "everyone plays music. After we gather to make music together, we can talk about problems in our community and how to resolve them. But our instruments are old and falling apart. Without music, so will we."* (Weisman, 1995)

For most of human history, music was essential to the communication and sense of connection within a tribe or village and was deeply integrated into the rituals, ceremonies, and celebrations that related to the deepest needs of the community. The current belief that music is primarily entertainment to be enjoyed separately from life's more serious obligations dominates contemporary culture with musical "product" such as recordings, videos, and concert performances all produced by professionals within the highly lucrative entertainment industry. The prevailing perception of music as basically a form of recreation permeates our society all the way through to our health and rehabilitation institutions. According to Anthony Salerno, founder of numerous residential rehabilitation centers:

> *The fact is, the vast majority of people who work in our profession, not to mention the clients, families, advocates, regulators, policy makers, legislators, elected and appointed officials, and the community at large—too often think of music therapy as only a recreational activity and they regard recreational activity as a method of residents keeping occupied. The fact that this belief is endemic is disturbing, but factual.* (personal communication, October 24, 2007)

Music therapists who work within recreation departments of institutions may be expected to facilitate large groups, making it difficult to establish an authentic alliance with many, if not most, clients. It is possible the music therapist may consciously or unconsciously align more with the needs of the institution than the needs of the client by seeing a lot of clients, doing a nice job on the paperwork, increasing the visibility of music in the facility, attempting to generate an appearance of "fun," and generally making things "look good" from an outward perception. One problem in determining what is, and is not, music therapy is that, in my experience, even under the worst conditions from a traditional therapy perspective, music is still a generally positive and uplifting experience for most clients in rehabilitation programs and institutional settings.

Music makes people feel good. We *play* music, and so it may appear inconsistent with the principles of serious work. Psychologist, linguist, and popular author Stephen Pinker (1997) dubbed music "auditory cheesecake" because, obviously, people liked it, but it didn't seem important or necessary to him. He could discern no survival benefit from mankind's universal and enduring practice of it. From my perspective, if something lasts from the dawn of humanity to the present day, it's important. That our prehistoric ancestors made music is clear, as evidenced by the discovery of bone flutes that are more than 50,000 years old (Tramo, 2001). I am sure music playing is much older than that. Music is deeply integrated into our neurology. The limbic system, an ancient part of the brain in evolutionary terms, has been demonstrated to be strongly responsive to music. This has led some researchers to conclude that music predates spoken language (Menon & Levitin, 2005). Brown (2001) proposed that early pre-language humans utilized a music language that conveyed information as well as emotional meaning using discrete pitch levels and expressive phrasing. Eventually, what Brown termed "Musilanguage" would split into two specialties, music and spoken language.

THE SOCIOPOLITICAL IMPETUS OF MUSIC THERAPY

Music therapy, by definition, endeavors to facilitate progress in the client, but does it also encourage cultural movement? Benzon (2001) hypothesized that music continues to play the role it did in humankind's beginning, what he called the forge in which the new forms of social being emerge. Music's "ripple effect"—its tendency to spread outward, naturally attract people and move them into increasingly wider social contexts (Pavlicevic & Ansdell, 2005)—is an integral aspect of music's nature, making it a natural vehicle for reflecting and challenging social boundaries. The Civil Rights Movement anthem, "We Shall Overcome," Bob Marley's "Redemption Song," Bob Dylan's "Blowing in the Wind," John Lennon's "Imagine," Woody Guthrie's "This Land Is Your Land"—these are popular songs that truly influenced the way people thought.

Music reflects its era as it illuminates the future and stretches social boundaries. In the Middle Ages, the Church restricted the use of certain harmonies that are now common. In the nineteenth century, the Waltz, and the dance it inspired, were considered immoral. Music and culture moved on, and these examples seem quaint by today's standards. In the twentieth century, the music of Stravinsky, avant-garde experimentation, jazz, rock, and rap were all met with resistance, outrage, and attempts at censorship. All these forms advanced the prevailing musical vocabulary and social culture in their day and are now integrated.

When I have been successful in establishing a strong music therapy program in an institution, it always had an effect on the internal culture. Musicologist Christopher Small (1998) claimed that all music is ultimately a political act, and music therapist Oksana Zharinova-Sanderson (2005) referred to the music therapist as a "campaigner for music as a force for change in the community" (p. 245). In one community music therapy program, of the multitude of original compositions, performances, and recordings we did in the facility, the head administrator would often say in staff meetings, "Once you hear the patients do this, you'll never view them the same way again." As a result, there was more respect and less condescension in staff-to-patient relationships.

Many individuals with lifelong disabilities such as mental illness, autism, intellectual disability, dementia, severe physical impairments, brain injury, and neurological disorders tend to spend most of their time in sheltered environments, such as therapeutic programs or schools, residences, or institutions. Since music therapists work to a large degree in these settings (AMTA, 2006), we may consider this question: "Where is the need for healing greater—in the individual with a disability or in the social conditions within which the disabled person resides?"

LOVE ME FOR WHO I AM

The following song, titled "Love Me for Who I Am," was written during one session in an in-patient residential institution. There were about 12 participants in this group and all had some form or another of significant impairment: brain injury, spinal cord injury, psychiatric diagnosis, orientation impairment, or memory disorder. Some could barely speak. Some barely knew where they were. Some were in wheelchairs. Some were grievously injured and not too physically attractive. A germ of an idea started about a better world. People started throwing out lines and suggestions. My job was to listen; to give everyone the respect of being heard and having a voice, even those whose voice was one word, a whisper, a hesitantly articulated contribution from a seemingly disoriented person who doesn't expect anyone to listen. As we fit the pieces together, little by little, a lyric took form. One lady who could play piano pretty well came up with some chords and a melody, a lilting calypso feel, maybe something like Harry Belafonte's "Jamaica Farewell." Suddenly, we had a song. Could any song be more socially significant and have a more timeless message?

Love Me for Who I Am

I may not look like you
I may not talk like you
But I have feelings
And my heart beats like you

If you take a little time
Then you might find
If you get to know me
You might come to love me

Though ages may pass
It must come at last
When the lion lies down with the lamb

The miracle is revealed
And the world will be healed
When you can love me for who I am

Ashes to ashes
Dust to dust
Life is risky
But in God we trust

Sadness will continue
To play its game
Until we realize
That we're all the same

Though ages may pass
It must come at last
When the lion lies down with the lamb

The miracle is revealed
And the world will be healed
When you can love me for who I am

"We have a right to be here. Our perspective is valid and our lives matter. We will not be condemned or pushed into the shadows." This is the heart of any social advocacy movement. The human tendency to split people into groups, with one group being the dominant and the other being the oppressed, has occurred throughout history, sometimes with monstrous results. Has any member of these groups been less capable or morally inferior to another? The dominant group at the time would try to make it seem so, but is it true?

GENIUS, PROPHET, PATIENT

Each individual, no matter what level of skills or IQ or social abilities, can become a contributing member of the community. This is what will give meaning to their lives.

—Dr. Temple Grandin, scientist, autism advocate (2011)

Rather than think of people with disabilities as being totally dependent, or, at best, having them fit in doing marginal work such as folding laundry in an institution or bagging groceries in a supermarket, could it be possible to include them as contributors in a society that values them for their strengths? "Everybody is a genius. But if you judge a fish by its ability to climb a tree, it will live its whole life believing that it is stupid" (attributed to Einstein, although it appears he did not actually say it). On the Autistic Self Advocacy Network website, it says:

The disability rights perspective within the Autistic community is represented in the neuro-diversity movement, which promotes social acceptance of neurological difference as part of the broad landscape of human diversity and seeks to bring about a world in which Autistic people enjoy the same access, rights, and opportunities as all other citizens. Acceptance of difference is essential to understanding, accepting, and benefiting from the contributions of everyone in our society, thus allowing all people to live up to their potential.

Of the seemingly dichotomous philosophies of "pulling oneself up by one's bootstraps" vs. "a civilized society that must care for its most vulnerable," neither is satisfactory. Many people cannot self-advocate and, at the same time, they don't just need care. Is it possible that some people who appear unable to make a contribution can actually have significant capabilities, some even beyond those of most people? Take Ronnie, for example, who will be discussed later: a completely dependent young man with no functional role in day-to-day society. Nonverbal with severe behavioral symptoms of autism, he is also a jigsaw puzzle genius. He doesn't even need to see the picture on the box. He is able to rapidly identify the shape of a piece and determine where it goes, completing the puzzle at a much faster pace and more efficiently than the best typical puzzle aficionado. What else could he do besides puzzles with this brilliance for visual-spatial processing—some type of advanced technical or engineering work? Is he incapable or is he oppressed because he's different? Does he have anything to offer? I've heard it said that people with disabilities (as we call them) are messengers. Is that simply idle talk?

DANIEL: HEAVEN AND EARTH

I will lead the blind by ways they have not known, along unfamiliar paths I will guide them; I will turn the darkness into light before them and make the rough places smooth. These are the things I will do; I will not forsake them.

—Isaiah 42:16

The first thing the reader needs to know is that, in every other case story in this book, I have changed people's names. In this story, the central individuals' actual names are used and the reason for this is beyond astounding. I will explain later.

When Daniel first came to the studio with his adopted mother, Patti, it was immediately clear he loved music very much and had an innate talent. Daniel was 25 years old and blind, as well as carrying a few other diagnoses including autism, obsessive compulsive disorder, and Tourette's syndrome. Although verbally fluent, he would not engage in a typical back-and-forth dialogue. His speech was full of nonsequiturs, seemingly free-associated comments and would cut off the thread of discussion at any time, saying, "I don't want to talk about it." He also engaged in some self-harm, hitting or biting himself, sometimes causing superficial, but not serious, injury. After striking himself, he would ask in a friendly, amused voice, "Now what am I doing? I'm hitting myself with my . . . what?" I was supposed to answer, "fist," but I soon learned not to encourage this. Patti said Daniel listened to the radio constantly and could play a little piano. At his first music therapy session, he sat down at the piano and began requesting song after song, mostly "oldie" rock songs or standard folk songs. He would not sing, although Patti said he sang at home. However, he could instantly locate the tonic on the piano, and he played insistent eighth notes on that one key throughout the song while I sang and played guitar. It was clear he knew hundreds of songs and, as one song was coming to an end, before the last line or two, he was already blurting out his next request.

Over time, I tried to help Daniel to calm down his frenetic approach, asking that we come to the end of one song before he suggested another. I taught him to play a two-note chord instead of one note but he kept on hitting the staccato eighth-notes so that he played every song in a driving style, reminiscent of early rock and roll. He could play a strong basic beat on a drum, and as he continued to improve on piano, he learned to play some left-hand bass lines, and soon he was soon picking out the melody of any song. He could do this effortlessly and immediately, without any practice. He also became willing to sing certain songs, and his pitch and rhythmic phrasing were excellent.

Hallelujah

It quickly became apparent how valuable this music time was for Daniel, particularly in contrast to the mind-numbing and condescending treatment in the day program he'd been attending. So Patti began bringing him multiple times during the week. For one of these sessions, I teamed Daniel up with a few other clients who came to the studio, two young men with whom he developed material and occasionally played concerts in supportive settings. During another session, he would regularly play with Melinda, a young woman with autism who came for her session after him. Melinda was an extraordinarily talented singer, and we usually did a few numbers together before Daniel left, notably, "Over the Rainbow," Leonard Cohen's "Hallelujah," and a few others. Patti would listen from the waiting room. One day, when her husband was in the hospital, an enormously stressful and heartbreaking situation (more on this in a moment), Patti sent me a message prior to the session: "I need to hear Daniel and you play 'Hallelujah' so bad today."

As it turned out, Patti couldn't make it to the session, so I asked Daniel's sister, Alice, who brought him, to film it on her phone with Melinda singing and Daniel on the piano. That evening, Patti sent me the following email:

Rick,

I just came home from the hospital after spending the day with my husband and I cannot tell you how much this video and recording means to me. I'll take it to the hospital tomorrow and play to Peter and he'll be over the moon happy. I explained to him this morning that Alice was with Daniel for music and we hoped to record the song. The video makes it the best. Thank you so very much. Such a ray of sunshine!

The following day, Patti and her husband watched the recording in the hospital numerous times. It lifted his spirits so to see Daniel participating in such a meaningful way, bringing joy to an unbearable situation.

Music therapy has become such an important part of Daniel's life, connecting him with other people, offering an opportunity to develop and be appreciated for his talents. Patti says he is always excited to come to music sessions. He is capable of the most infectious joy when we are working on something that excites him. His musical gift continues to unfold as he plays more and more challenging pieces and his ability to stay focused and collaborate also progresses. Patti feels he lives in a musical world, but it was previously mostly a private world. Now he's sharing it.

According to Patti, "His whole world has opened up. You can't possibly understand what you are accomplishing through your efforts. Music has helped Daniel to find himself through the adversity and handicapping of his autism, OCD, Tourette's and total darkness in blindness. Music truly has given him the gift of life."

* * *

While Daniel's musical gift is wonderful enough in enriching his life, there are other gifts he has to share. Daniel was born to a poor, unwed mother in an Asian country. Given up at birth, he resided in an orphanage under deplorable conditions. He was strapped into a crib and left by himself for most of the day with no attention other than the minimum feeding or cleaning—no interaction, no stimulation, no play, no toys. Patti said that these underprivileged, discarded babies were simply left to die. Daniel is blind because he was born with congenital glaucoma that would have been easily curable with treatment. However, it was not addressed at all, no care, no medication. A representative from a U.S. adoption agency that traveled worldwide seeking such abandoned, disabled, but possibly adoptable children, spotted an eighteen-month-old Daniel attempting to amuse himself with a shiny object that must have fallen into his crib. He was passing it back and forth in front of his one eye that still retained a slight capability to discern flickers of light. The representative thought maybe the boy still possessed just enough spirit and playfulness to be adoptable and so brought him back to the United States.

Luckily for Daniel, he came to the attention of Patti and Peter, a couple that had adopted a number of children with significant challenges. Patti and Peter were told by doctors that Daniel could not be expected to talk. But also luckily for Daniel, Patti and Peter had an eleven-year-old biological son, Peter Jr., who took an interest in Daniel. Peter Jr. was not blind but he was also visually impaired, and he wanted to help Daniel. Peter Jr. and Daniel became very close. Contrary to the experts' prognosis, Daniel did learn to talk although he appeared internally preoccupied, frequently talking to himself and making strange, non-sequitur statements. Still, he was a friendly, social, spirited child, and he went to a school that served children with special needs. People seemed to like him and to be drawn to him, but Peter Jr. remained his closest relationship.

Then, when Daniel was 10, Peter Jr. suddenly and tragically died of an aneurysm. Although Patti and Peter Sr. were devastated, Daniel did not appear to be. Patti noticed him talking to himself, which wasn't out of the ordinary, but it seemed conversational, as if he was listening and responding. When his mother asked him about it, Daniel said he was talking to Peter Jr. This was very hard for Patti to handle as she was in deep grief over the loss and, in any case, she wasn't too sure what she believed about life after death and people communicating with the dead. Daniel would tell Patti things Peter Jr. said such as, "Don't cry, I'm still here." This may not sound too convincing for skeptics, but Patti also said that sometimes Daniel would ask her questions based on information he couldn't have possibly known, saying Peter Jr. told him about it. If asked about Peter Jr., Daniel would speak about him in a matter-of-fact manner, as if he was right there or was away at the moment and would be back soon just like any family member at work or school. One Christmas morning, Patti was sitting on the couch and Daniel came over and said, "Move over Peter. I want to sit next to Mommy." "I couldn't handle that one," said Patti.

Patti and Peter Sr. prepared Daniel for life ahead by enrolling him in a residential school for the blind. The school also reported that Daniel would sit in his room and talk to himself and, when asked about it, would say he was talking to Peter Jr. Daniel became very close to his primary instructor at the school, Kenneth. Daniel said Peter Jr. told him that Kenneth had a purple front door at his house. What a person, blind since birth, would know about "purple" was one question to consider, but Kenneth confirmed that it was indeed the case. (Later, Daniel was to tell me that Peter Jr. told him I had a brick fireplace in my house, which was also true.)

Daniel graduated at age 18, having learned essential skills about navigating the world as a blind person, but when he returned home, there wasn't too much for him to do. He was an energetic, happy young man, but because of his unconventional behavior, verbal outbursts, talking to himself, self-involvement and so forth, he couldn't be expected to hold any type of regular job. His mother took him to day programs, swimming lessons, sports programs, horseback riding, and eventually, music.

As it turned out, Peter Jr. wasn't the only deceased person with whom Daniel was in communication. When Daniel told Patti that Gerri told him Joan (Daniel's swimming instructor) needed help, Patti didn't know what he could mean or who Gerri was. When Patti asked Joan about it, Joan broke down crying, saying that Gerri was her deceased sister. Joan then explained that she was in emotional turmoil—overwhelmed, depressed, and lonely taking care of her invalid father and struggling with indecision as to whether she should adopt a child.

Daniel's gift has touched my life as well. One day when Patti brought Daniel in for his session, she said on the way he kept saying over and over, "I have a message for Rick." When I asked what that message might be, he said, in his typical manner, "I don't know." However, when pressed by Patti, he finally said, "Dottie loves Lise." That's it; no further elaboration. Dottie is my deceased mother, and Lise is my sister, people I had never mentioned to Daniel. When I told this story to Lise, she began to weep. She said that very week she had been experiencing a profound wave of grief over the loss of our parents eight years prior and was reading a book by a renowned psychic that outlined methods to communicate with the deceased. She was trying, without success, some of the techniques in the book, seeking a connection, a message of some kind. Through Daniel, our mother found a way to console her, to express her enduring love.

Another example occurred a few months after that. I was climbing a mountainous rockface with my son. About halfway up, I realized it was more difficult and dangerous than I first realized and there was a potential for either me or my son to have a serious fall. As I paused on a precipice and negotiated my impending panic, I realized there was nothing to do but go on, so I took a deep breath and continued. Everything worked out fine, although I was a little shaken up. The next day, Patti told me that during the time I was on the ledge, Daniel had blurted out (inexplicably for her at that moment), "Dottie is afraid Rick is going to fall."

Daniel began passing along other messages to me from deceased loved ones. He told me that my father and uncle were happy with their mother. He told me my grandparents were together and loved me. These weren't vague statements. He used their names; names of people I never referred to in any way; some of them uncommon Russian-Jewish names. There are other examples too uncanny to be happenstance. Daniel can never elaborate or answer follow-up questions beyond his initial statements. "You have to understand," said Patti, "these are things he hears. He doesn't know what they mean."

Then, as alluded to above, tragedy struck again in Daniel's family. Peter Sr. was diagnosed with advanced terminal cancer. As Peter's condition rapidly deteriorated, Daniel repeatedly told Patti, "Peter say one, two, nine. Peter say one, two, nine." When asked what he meant, Daniel said, "I don't know." Patti couldn't figure it out. Peter Sr. passed away on January 29, 1/29. Patti was devastated. Peter had been her childhood sweetheart and they'd been together for over fifty years. Daniel expressed no sense of loss. As when Peter Jr., passed, Daniel would say to Patti, "Daddy say 'Don't cry.'"

I Got You, Babe

Patti wanted to maintain Daniel's normal routine as much as possible and so continued to send him to music. During the weeks following Peter Sr.'s passing, Daniel was brought by his older sister, Alice, who lived in Europe but had come home for a while to help out. One day, Daniel and I were having fun with the Sonny and Cher song, "I Got You, Babe." As you may know, the song is a duet with Sonny and Cher taking alternating lines in the verse and singing together in the chorus. Daniel and I had worked on this song before with Daniel taking one part and me taking the other, but Daniel was often inconsistent, sometimes singing his line at the proper time, sometimes not, sometimes losing concentration, sometimes mumbling his lines in a distracted way. From a music-therapy-goal point of view, one might say the song offered a good way to work on Daniel's confidence, sense of collaboration and focus.

On this occasion, I discovered if we sat right next to each other and Daniel held a microphone while I sometimes held his hand holding the mic, I could casually direct the way the mic was pointing, toward my mouth when it was my turn or toward his mouth for his line. Daniel responded to this cue and subtle motivational technique, pulling off a perfect rendition of the song. A music therapy intern accompanied on guitar so that I could focus on singing with Daniel. We tried it a second time, and I asked Alice to make a video of us on her phone to show Patti. Videos of Daniel's music always filled her with joy, and I thought this might give her a moment's respite from her overwhelming grief. The next day I received the following note from Patti:

Rick,

I think I have played the "I've Got You Babe" video about 50 times since Alice brought Daniel home yesterday. The County Health nurse came to visit yesterday and she watched the video and cried with me! Daniel even sat on our couch with the nurse and sang some of his favorite songs that he does with you. It was amazing to watch him. He enjoyed performing for her so much. When he finished he told the nurse "Daddy say he's happy!" So it's started already. He's giving me messages from his Dad and I know it's all meant to be. I'm sure Peter's spirit is here and I'm sure he enjoyed this video as much as he did the one you did for him while he was in the hospital.

It's golden Rick. In the midst of so much grief you have given us this most precious inspiration. I won't give up. Daniel inspires me enough to want to live and keep going.

Best, Patti

This is what it's all about for me. Music's capacity to lighten unbearable pain, to inspire, to connect, to counter despair, to extend outward—through Daniel to Alice to Patti to the nurse to who knows whom else if the nurse told someone about it. A few moments of music, inconsequential, even trivial, to the world at large, touch and uplift the lives of multiple people.

Now, as to why I use the actual names of Daniel, Patti, Peter Sr., and Peter Jr., as opposed to pseudonyms, as I mentioned at the top of this chapter. Patti told me that the day before one of our sessions, Daniel was being excessively chatty; going on and on about me: "When are we going to see Rick? Is it music time tomorrow? Is it going to rain? I don't want it to rain. Will we still see Rick if it rains? . . ." He was also talking about (and possibly to) his father when he said: "Daddy says tell Rick, Peter not Paul." Patti had no idea what that might mean when she mentioned it to me. Then she asked Daniel again when he came to music, "What did Daddy say to Rick?" Daniel reiterated, "Daddy says, Peter, not Paul." After a moment's thought, my jaw hit the floor. Originally, as I was writing this chapter, I had used the name Paul as a pseudonym for Peter Sr. I also changed Patti's name to Peggy and Daniel's to Randall. I could only think that Peter Sr. wanted me to use his actual name in the recounting of this story! If this interpretation is correct, the implications are staggering. It would mean that Peter was somehow aware of my thoughts, his name change existing only in my mind (and on my computer) at that point!

One more story—Daniel walked into Patti's bedroom at 3 a.m. and woke her up to tell her that Daddy was there and he was talking to her. In the morning, Daniel told Patti that Daddy was still there and he was saying, "Happy Anniversary." At first that made no sense to Patti. Their wedding anniversary was months away until Patti realized that the day was, in fact, the anniversary of their first date together fifty years ago!

If one believes Daniel's gift to see beyond this mortal coil holds credence, then it is clear he has much to offer, answering some of the deepest questions of humanity and comforting the troubled. He has certainly provided some solace to Patti through her agonizing losses. But my acceptance of the genuineness of Daniel's extraordinary capabilities come not only from Patti's anecdotes. His imparting of messages to me from deceased family members, mentioning names that he could not know by any stretch of the imagination, constitutes indisputable evidence of the life of spirit after death. What does Patti think about all this? We have frequent conversations, and she often follows up with further thoughts in an email. Following one of these conversations, she wrote this:

I believe that Daniel was put in my life for a very distinct purpose. I most likely will never live to comprehend the entire sanctity of the true passage

> *he presents to me. Then I say it matters not to analyze and purport into my interruptions. I don't feel that's important. Others have said it's too bad Daniel is hindered by his blindness and his spectrums. Imagine, they say, how talented he could have become. To know Daniel as I do, I say he's perfect just the way he is. The real beauty in Daniel's spirit is not in what he could have been or could have produced. Daniel's beauty is in the message he's attempting to show this world of cookie cutter persons that he is beyond all those expectations. His gift with music is showing us the comfort and absolute resolve a human finds in being lifted with such an exhilaration it soars to unimaginable heights. There is no psychological therapy or drug therapy to release the mind into utopia that music therapy can give us. I find this so evident just to witness Daniel enjoy his time with you exploring more and more of his world. I treasure each session I can attend with him to give me the feeling that life ultimately does give us goodness and to celebrate each day.*
>
> *In conclusion, I believe Daniel connects to you, Rick, as you are the direct link to his uncultured talent. Daniel is as a funnel to the spiritual world. The souls on the other side are drawn to this funnel as a port to interrupt unseen to most in this world. Because you are key to his purpose many will speak to you through him. You are unique in your abilities to find the gifts of the disadvantaged and to display these gifts on the world's stage in life. You possess a genius undercurrent to again relate what is unseen by much of life.*
>
> *Daniel had come into our lives as a messenger to try to heal, if you may, some of the abomination that is around us in daily life. Life is in need of direction right now. How many will possibly understand the disadvantaged give us insight to the gift of peace?* (personal communication, October 1, 2020)

For those who remain skeptical, I can only offer this quote by Shakespeare from *Hamlet*:

> *There are more things in heaven and earth, Horatio,*
> *Than are dreamt of in your philosophy.*

THE ORIGIN OF CONSCIOUSNESS IN THE BREAKDOWN OF THE BICAMERAL MIND

> *"You're sick! Don't you understand that? You're sick! You can't just do whatever you want. You have to do what I tell you because you're sick!"*

While working in the psychiatric department at a large New York City hospital, I overheard the above statement emanating from a psychiatrist's office as he angrily berated a patient (who I would assume was being noncompliant with his medication). It is not an exact quotation because it happened a long time ago but that was the gist of it. I remember the doctor yelling and he called the patient sick, numerous times. I don't know if the doctor's strategy worked or not, but either way it sounded like abuse to me.

Mental, emotional, and behavioral problems are not the same as a broken leg in terms of clarity of diagnosis and treatment. Neuro-researchers have been unable to find any evidence to support the breakdown of mental characteristics into separate diagnostic categories as defined in the American Psychiatric Association's influential *Diagnostic and Statistical Manual of Mental Disorders* (Adam, 2103). "Once you label me you negate me," said Kierkegaard (Vriend & Dyer, 1976). Even if some psychiatrists and neuroscientists would like to claim that all human behavior can be explained in terms of neural functioning that can be identified, this logic doesn't differentiate between which behavior would require medication and which behavior is okay. This is simply a matter of opinion, isn't it? Some might say the psychiatrist in the above example could use some medication. In the Music Therapy Studio, I accept people at face value. To more medically oriented people who lean toward the disease model and might think my approach is naive or inconsequential, I would say I guess we all have our place. But it is helpful to be open to other views.

Speaking of other views, a best-selling but controversial book from the seventies by Dr. Julian Jaynes, the title of which is the name of this section, proposed that ancient people experienced the world in a manner that has similarities to schizophrenia. This book was very influential to me when I first read it in shifting my thinking from the disease model to a broader way of considering what is characterized as pathology. Jayne's contention was that rather than making conscious evaluations, these earlier people literally heard advice or direction similar to auditory hallucinations without being aware of their own thought processes. As societies shifted further into the current cognitively based, problem-solving form of consciousness, those who heard voices were considered mad. For those individuals, now misunderstood, dismissed, diagnosed, treated, institutionalized, and tormented by shame, the voices would turn negative, perhaps mocking or asserting that one was no good or commanding one to kill oneself.

Obviously, some people discounted Jaynes's theory, but it was a scholarly work and was not altogether dismissed. Further research in the late nineties using brain imaging technology brought renewed acknowledgment to Jaynes's ideas for contributing to a rethinking of auditory hallucinations and mental illness (Smith, 2007). There is no doubt that people do hear voices. Is it purely a disorder or could it have other antecedents?

I have worked with many people diagnosed as schizophrenic and have often found them to be sensitive, occasionally exceptional individuals. Some people diagnosed with schizophrenia do seem to have disordered or confused thought patterns, but others seem reasonably lucid except they hear voices or see things that others don't perceive. I am positively convinced that there are objective phenomena beyond the realm of sensory perception, so I am open to the idea that some perception dismissed as hallucinatory is absolutely real. I am not taking an indisputable position. I'm just saying I am open. I can recall occasions when people with schizophrenia displayed extraordinary sensitivities that seemed to approach the extrasensory. Scoff if you must. I take Jaynes's theory simply as food for thought that I can neither prove nor disprove. However, if I have to misjudge people, I'd rather err on the side of counting them in rather than counting them out.

Sometimes, people with schizophrenia can be tortured souls. It must be terrifying to have hallucinations and be labeled a sick person who needs to be normalized. I'm all for helping people who are suffering if it is possible, but often medications and institutions can't really change the basic profile of a person that much. They might mute some of the more intense symptoms or provide some supportive services. But still, the person is who he or she is. Whatever works in helping someone to have a better life is admirable. My point is in respecting each person for the gifts they may have and integrating them even if they do not fit into the prevailing social framework. Some people are not going to "get better." They simply are the way they are. It will be a long time before society catches up with this idea, but in the Music Therapy Studio we don't need to wait for society. We can lead the way, and we can start right now.

NOEL: TO MAKE A BETTER WORLD FOR *ALL* TO SEE

Noel walked into my studio with a support staff person, sat down at the piano, and began to play. I immediately realized I was in the presence of an exceptional talent. He ran one song into the next—pop to classical to gospel—playing with confidence and command, using complex harmonies, shifting keys effortlessly. He was also obviously quite eccentric, gesturing strangely, seemingly talking to people that I didn't see, verbalizing all types of nonsequiturs and disorganized flight of ideas. I assumed he had been diagnosed with some form of schizophrenia, but when I later spoke to his brother, he was unwilling to call it that, saying that Noel had been labeled with so many diagnoses over the years, there was no point in calling it one thing or another. He simply explained that Noel, now age 64, developed a profound thought-disorganization sometime in late adolescence, leading to a lifetime of disability. Noel was friendly, respectful, and communicative, but often mumbled, said incomprehensible things, and displayed a constant fidgety, nervous energy.

He rushed through songs and played quite powerfully, almost pounding at times, but his musical gift was unmistakable. He said he wanted me to be his piano instructor and teach him Brahms, Bach, Schubert—a bit of a problem, since not only did I not have much of a classical repertoire, but Noel's ability on the piano far exceeded mine. I couldn't teach him anything about the piano. I did see how I could help him to focus, collaborate, settle down a bit, get his gift a little more under control, and feel acknowledged and appreciated for the excellent musician he was.

Playing along with him on guitar or bass or sometimes singing, I helped him to play at a more moderate tempo, without breaking off or veering unexpectedly into something else, and to stay together with me, rather than rushing ahead on his own. We started to develop some mutual repertoire. A little before Christmas, we made a set list of holiday songs and did a few volunteer gigs at a local nursing home. Noel was a great success, being much appreciated by both residents and administration. The difference between Noel on piano—steady, engaged, brilliant—and Noel off the piano—a mass of gesticulations and unintelligible comments to no one in particular—was striking.

Whatever his diagnosis was, it made no difference to me. My interest was in Noel the musician and in establishing trust and alliance. After Christmas, we began to prepare a new set of non-holiday songs to continue playing out. The focus, sharing, and appreciation of his musical gift in a public setting had seemed to be very beneficial to him. One day as we were rehearsing, Noel suddenly introduced a song he said he had written: a beautiful anthemic ballad with sophisticated harmonies. He sang the following lyrics:

Faith, Hope, Love, Joy
Mercy, Grace, Peace, Patience
Truth, Nobility, Life, Light
Faith, Hope, Love, Joy

And we live our life
And we think our thoughts
And we mention what is friendly

And we live our life
And we think our thoughts
Each and every day

In the Bible
There's revival
And it talks of things like love and peace and joy
And happiness
To make a better world for everyone to see

Hallelujah Ecstasy Fantasy Reality
Decency Dignity Thoughtfulness. Consideration
Marvelous. Magnificent. Miraculous. Astounding
Amazing Divine Joy

I was taken aback as this stunning Baroque/Gospel-influenced composition unfolded before me; astonished that this fellow, so psychologically disturbed in one way, was capable of this. The composition's basic structure was founded in standard I - VI - IV - V Ionian chord changes, but then there were some surprising chromatic shifts that revealed a sophisticated musical mind at work. Every word in the opening stanzas featured a different chord change that gave weight and emphasis to each spiritual trait, and the list in the last stanza shifted tempos and also had a different chord-change for each word. I knew Noel attended a Christian church regularly, and although his lyric referred to the Bible, it was not dogmatic, proselytizing, nor did it mention Jesus. It sounded like early Christian philosophy before it was established by the Church but it could have been Old Testament, for that matter. It simply contained the non-judgmental and universal message inherent in all religions and spiritual thought: living together in peace and love.

Call me a romantic, but I had never heard Noel play anything like this before, and as his song poured forth in front of me, I felt as if I was receiving a pure message of truth from a great soul. Calling him a prophet might be hyperbolic, but that's how it felt in the moment. There was nothing self-centered about it, no agenda to convince anyone of anything or even particularly to be appreciated. Just beautiful music and a lone voice of truth in the wilderness, there for one to listen to or not, to put one's own meaning on it or ignore it completely, like a sunset, the stars at night, or a child's smile. Where in the world is there a place for Noel's song to be heard, developed, and esteemed for its grandeur and timeless message? In the Music Therapy Studio. Who will join in with his song? I will.

But then I thought, perhaps it could be more than just me appreciating his song. Songs are meant to be shared. I thought we could get a group of people together to sing Noel's song. I asked Noel if he liked the idea, and he did. We began rehearsing with a few music therapy students. One problem, I initially thought, was that Noel kept tagging the chorus of the huge eighties pop phenomenon, "We Are the World," on at the end of his song as a medley. While I could see how it fit musically and thematically, I thought his song should be wholly original and attempted to persuade him to do something else. There was another chord sequence he often played, and I tried to help him write some lyrics. Noel went along with me, but he rarely played it correctly, and, in any case, it felt like it didn't belong there. Then we tried to adapt a gospel standard as a chorus outro, but that also felt forced and incorrect.

The whole thing was basically an exercise in frustration, and after several sessions of trying to complete his song, Noel walked into the studio and laid down the law. We can do anything except work on his song. It seemed he was tired of having me push him to take his song in a different direction than his original conception, and in any case, I don't think he saw the point of all this trouble. We just jammed that session and played whatever he wanted. Nevertheless, when I asked him, Noel replied that he still retained interest in the idea of singing his song with a group of people. I know when I'm licked, so "We Are the World" it was for the outro.

I invited a few music therapy students and a few other clients who liked to sing to join us, and I arranged a date with the local assisted living facility where we had previously played for all of us to gather and sing Noel's song. Noel continued to express positivity for the project, but the week before it was scheduled to take place, as we tried to rehearse, Noel was erratic. He kept veering off into other songs and playing at inconsistent tempos. We couldn't get it together, and I wondered if the whole thing was a mistake. What if I got all these people together to sing Noel's song and he didn't want to play it or he played in a way that was impossible to follow?

I did discover one technique that worked. If I sat right next to Noel and played my guitar while he played his piano, I found we locked in on the changes and tempo more effectively. We ran through the song one time successfully this way and Noel seemed done. I realized I couldn't push him any further. The rehearsal was arduous for him, so I backed off and we played whatever he wanted for the remainder of the session.

After the rehearsal session, I deliberated. Should we even do this? What was the point? Was I setting Noel and everybody else up for a disorienting, disappointing experience? Was this simply my grand ambition and not in his interest at all? I thought about it for a few days and talked to a few colleagues. I decided to take a chance. No guts, no glory. Nevertheless, I prepared a Plan B. Plan A was to film and record everybody singing his song. However, if Noel couldn't organize himself enough to rehearse and do a few takes to get a nice rendition, I would just discard the whole idea. Plan B was to let him do a piano bar-style sing-along. Noel knew a lot of songs, and I was fairly sure that would go well. It had gone well before. Only I and the music therapy students would be the wiser. Everyone would have a reasonably good time. We'd get in and get out. Nobody would get hurt.

On the appointed day, we assembled at the facility. About ten residents wanted to participate as singers. Others watched. Three other clients and four music therapy students showed up to sing. We arranged ourselves in choir fashion, with one student acting as conductor and Noel and me sitting right next to each other in the back, me on acoustic guitar, Noel on piano. Take One: Noel played beautifully, with restraint, precision, feeling. The residents and clients learned the song. Take Two—pretty good. Let's try one more. Take Three: In the can. Noel's playing was consistent and perfect throughout: a true master. All the struggle and worry had no relevance to this situation. The assisted living home residents loved the song. One said she wanted to take it to her church choir to see if they would sing it. Noel, as well as everyone else, felt uplifted, invigorated, and competent—as successful an event as could be expected!

Noel's dominant life as an isolated person with a psychiatric disability was nowhere to be found. While it might be an exaggeration to call Noel a genius, he certainly has a great talent. And on this day, he did what those with great talents do: he raised his game to meet the situation and, in the process, took us all with him, inspiring us and offering a glimpse of the better world that his song embodied.

3

Sacred Space

The musical space is a contained space. It is an intimate and private field created in the relationship between the therapist and client. It is a sacred space which becomes identified as 'home base,' a territory which is well known and secure.

—*Carolyn Kenny, music therapist (1989)*

THE MUSIC ROOM

When we speak about the Music Therapy Studio space, of course we have in mind the physical environment—the look of the room, the setup of the room, the size of the room, the acoustics of the room, extraneous sounds outside the room. All these things can impact the quality of the musical experiences, but I don't believe we should be too precious about it. A music therapist cannot be a diva. Music therapy can be conducted anywhere: a hospital room, a rented room in a church, an institutional day room, a spare office. What matters is the sacred space created between therapist and client. I once conducted a music therapy session in a large, noisy day room in a city hospital. People were walking in and out. Some people were watching TV on the other side of the room, and maintenance men were working on the radiator. I don't know if you can call that a sacred space. I'll admit I wasn't too happy about it, but I did the best I could. That was where I was asked to do it, and that was where the patients were. They were either there with music or without it.

Different practitioners have different ideas about their physical space. Some music therapy rooms tend toward the clinical. There isn't much in them except perhaps a guitar or piano and a few instruments the therapist chooses to bring in for the client, perhaps a drum or small marimba or shaker. It might be thought that, particularly for children, too many options might lead to overwhelm and loss of focus

In my studio, all the instruments are in plain sight. I have never noticed it to be overstimulating, even for children with all sorts of issues such as sensory processing disorder, hyperactivity, impulse control problems, anxiety, aggression, or other behavior problems. They seem to simply gravitate toward that which interests them, and the rest of it doesn't seem to distract them. If they are going to have focus or impulse control issues, I think they are going to have them regardless of whether there are a few more instruments in the room or not. In the outside world, we need to be able to manage an unending stream of stimulation and not become overwhelmed. Why should a therapy room be so controlled? Is that learning how to manage in the world? I'm not making a case for a messy room, but to me the most important considerations are: Does this look like a place where people play music? Do I feel comfortable here? When people walk into my studio, does it communicate: Safety, Creativity, Open-Mindedness, Connection?

HOLDING SPACE

The concept referred to as "holding space" was designed primarily in relation to working with or relating to people going through traumatic circumstances, particularly dying or serious illness. It means that we are willing to walk alongside another person in whatever journey they're on with open hearts, letting go of judgment and control. To support people in their growth, transformation, or grief, it may be necessary to accept our own powerlessness to do anything other than be present.

We can't:

- fix the problem.
- discount the problem or feeling or make it go away.
- imply we know what to do.
- give unnecessary or unwanted advice.

We can:

- honor the situation and each person's way of dealing with it.
- allow clients to make their own choices.
- help clients to feel safe and supported.

- accept complex emotions.
- be present.

What is the music that can emerge from this space?

INTERACTIVE SPACE

The Tao does nothing, yet leaves nothing undone.
If powerful men and women
could center themselves in it,
the whole world would be transformed by itself,
in its natural rhythms.
People would be content
with their simple, everyday lives,
in harmony, and free of desire.

When life is simple, pretenses fall away;
our essential nature shines through.
When there is no desire, all things are at peace.

When there is silence,
one finds the anchor of the universe
within oneself

—*Tao te Ching, Verse 37*

Music therapist Gary Ansdell (1995) considers the interactive space created by the music makers to be the vital area where a "creative sharing of musical thought occurs" (p. 221), and where the relationship develops between client and therapist. The client "hears himself being heard and responds to his being responded to" (p. 69). How much of the interactive space is the therapist occupying with his or her agenda? This is an essential consideration. If we are overactive, filling up the situation with too much of our own music, beliefs, expectations, perhaps insecurities, where is the space for the client? If a music therapist is singing all the lyrics, playing their instrument continuously with full harmonies and the rhythm chugging along, where is the client's part? If there are any stops or moments of tension in the music where the therapist is hoping the client might fill in with a word or instrument, if the client doesn't do it fast enough, will the therapist do that, too? If it doesn't seem too important or compelling, the client may not participate. There's no space.

A music therapist may think it is important to be exciting, to play with intensity, or make a big sound, to inspire clients to join in, but it is actually sometimes just the opposite. Play less. Invite more. Clients may be dealing with endless messages from every other quarter of their lives that they can't do this or that; that they're not capable. Everyone around them is doing for them, compensating for their supposed incapacities. A client may be habituated to a degree of withdrawal or passivity. After all, the music therapist is the expert. Why bother? A practitioner might want IT to happen, "the real thing"; that magical moment where the client's growth becomes evident in some way, but there is no place for this expansion to take place.

Do we believe in the power of music? Can we create an interactive space where the absolute unshakable faith in the power of music is simply a given? Do we believe in the potential of our clients? The following quotation is often attributed to the poet e.e. cummings, although apparently, that is an error. It is from a book called *Please Touch* by Edwin M. Campbell and Peter A. McMahon (1976). In any case, it says a lot for the Music Therapy Studio:

> *We do not believe in ourselves until someone reveals that deep inside us something is valuable, worth listening to, worthy of our trust, sacred to our touch. Once we believe in ourselves we can risk curiosity, wonder, spontaneous delight or any experience that reveals the human spirit.*

To believe means to trust in something outside of what currently is. This is the essence of creativity. The Bible refers to "the substance of things hoped for, the evidence of things not seen" (Heb. 11:1). Our belief is the space our clients can occupy. Beliefs are the walls, the enclosure in which the real thing happens. We cannot make the real thing happen, but we can create the interactive space within which the real thing is allowed to happen.

AKASHA

> *We mold clay into a pot,*
> *but it is the emptiness inside*
> *that makes the vessel useful.*
> *We fashion wood for a house,*
> *but it is the emptiness inside*
> *that makes it livable.*
> *We work with the substantial,*
> *but the emptiness is what we use.*
>
> —*Tao te Ching, Verse 11*

The Sanskrit word Akasha, translated as both ether and space, refers to the subtlest vibratory element in the material world. According to physicist David Bohm (1980): "Space is not empty. It is full, a plenum as opposed to a vacuum, and is the ground for the existence of everything, including ourselves. The universe is not separate from this cosmic sea of energy."

From the perspectives of both the ancient Greek and Ayurvedic traditions, space is referred to as ether. It is the space the other elements—earth, water, fire, air—fill. In musical terms, we might (very generally) consider the elements this way (Bosco, 1992):

Earth	*Foundation*	*Bass/Pulse*
Water	*Flowing*	*Harmony*
Fire	*Propulsion*	*Rhythmic Parts*
Air	*Breath*	*Singing/Melody*

Nothing can exist without space. Ether is active, not empty space. Ether is an aspect of physical manifestation and the background against which the material universe becomes perceptible. Ether is the most expansive of the elements, without form, boundaries, or limits. Perhaps ether is thought: what we believe or don't believe (more on this in later chapters). What are we going to let in? When we enter a session, with what sounds, feelings, ideas, belief systems, do we fill it?

> *Painters paint their pictures on canvas. Musicians paint their pictures on silence.*
>
> *—Leopold Stokowski (1967)*

4

Lessons from Nordoff-Robbins

Paul Nordoff, award-winning composer, virtuoso pianist, and professor of music, and Clive Robbins, special education teacher, met in England in 1958. Following some early collaborative experiments with music and disabled children, they became so profoundly convinced of the power of music as therapy that they each gave up their former careers to pursue a working partnership. This ultimately led to international Nordoff-Robbins Centers, training programs, and coauthored books that outlined an approach and philosophy for music therapy that changed the field forever.

I've introduced some of the ideas of Nordoff-Robbins already and will continue to reference them throughout this book. Obviously, they have been enormously influential to me along with the work of notable Nordoff-Robbins–trained practitioners who followed in their footsteps, such as New York University's Dr. Alan Turry and Dr. Kenneth Aigen and the UK's Dr. Gary Ansdell, names you will also see pop up a fair amount. I would probably not have even made the transition into music therapy if it wasn't for these powerful role models. Most music therapy prior to Nordoff and Robbins was predisposed to behavioral approaches and remains so in many contemporary schools of thought. If I balked at the idea of referring to people as a clinical population, as I mentioned in my backstory, had I concluded that music therapy meant I was supposed to approach people using music as a reinforcer, determine target behaviors, and collect data from repeated measurements, I would have definitely headed for the hills, and perhaps this gray-bearded rocker would be playing "I Can't Get No Satisfaction" in some bar with a sawdust-covered floor tonight.

With their integration of reverence for music, searching philosophy, and painstakingly conscientious clinical methodology, the Nordoff-Robbins approach has attracted a multitude of astute clinicians, inspired countless students, and made an indispensable contribution to the field of music therapy. Barbara Hesser, who founded the music therapy program at New York University, wrote in the preface to the reissue of Nordoff and Robbins's first widely available book (originally published in 1971), *Therapy in Music for Handicapped Children* (2005): "At that time I did not find the music therapy clinical work that I saw or read about to be what I envisioned possible, and I was at a crossroads in my decision whether to continue in my pursuit of music therapy as a career. It was reading this book that confirmed my belief that the artistic and creative use of music was indeed a powerful tool for work with the mental, physical and emotional problems of children" (p. 7).

When I was first introduced to the ideas of Nordoff and Robbins in the early days of my studies at New York University, they deeply resonated with me. But I was a guitarist/singer with stylistic roots primarily in rock, folk, and blues, and, to me, Nordoff-Robbins was a pianist's world. The extraordinary command—both technically and clinically—in Paul Nordoff's classically influenced piano approach established a legacy so formidable as to appear practically impossible for a primary therapist to play in another style, let alone another instrument, and still call it Nordoff-Robbins music therapy. And, indeed, that was the way it stayed well into the nineties. Although I read the Nordoff-Robbins's literature and adopted many of the concepts as my own, I couldn't foresee any further in-depth study of the approach beyond my New York University master's degree.

That all changed in 2000 when, through a series of events that seemed somehow miraculous, I was offered a scholarship to become the third person to focus exclusively on guitar as a primary instrument during my certification training as a Nordoff-Robbins Music Therapist. To his credit as a progressive thinker, Clive seemed most enthusiastic about my involvement as a guitarist, illustrating another shining feature, which Hesser described: "One of the wonderful aspects of Nordoff-Robbins work is that it is dynamic and does not stay static. It is always evolving as each new generation of therapists adds its unique experience, understanding and talent" (p. 7). It was a life and mind-expanding experience to study with Clive Robbins and the staff at the New York Center.

So with all that in mind, let's look at some of the key concepts of Nordoff-Robbins Music Therapy.

THE MUSIC CHILD

> *The Music Child is the individualized musicality inborn in each child. The term has reference to the universality of musical sensitivity—the heritage of complex sensitivity to the ordering and relationship of tonal and rhythmic movement. It also points to the distinctly personal significance of each child's musical responsiveness. The concept is not limited to the child with special musical gifts but focuses attention on that entity in every child which responds to musical experience, finds it meaningful and engaging, remembers music, and enjoys some form of musical expression.*
>
> *—Nordoff and Robbins (1977, p. 1)*

The "Music Child" lies at the heart of the Nordoff-Robbins philosophy. Coined by Nordoff and Robbins (1977) in the early days of establishing their theoretical concepts, it is founded on the premise that humans are innately prepared to engage in and respond to music. The model of the "Music Child" illustrates how the boundaries of the "Condition Child" (the limited sense of self the child has developed in response to his or her particular disability) begin to expand as the child, through the inspiration and lead of the inner "Music Child," relates to himself and others in ways that were not previously manifest.

Nordoff and Robbins's early work was with children, which explains the specificity of the term. Today, Nordoff-Robbins–trained music therapists work with every age group. So perhaps we might update it to Music Person (*Homo Musicus*, meaning Musical Human, is a phrase Dr. Robbins would use often). The conviction is that music is not simply an activity people do. It is something all people *are*. To quote one of Nordoff-Robbins's early influences, mid-twentieth-century musicologist Viktor Zuckerkandl (1973), the Musical Person is a "being that requires music to realize itself fully" (p. 2). Nordoff-Robbins therapist and scholar Dr. Ken Aigen (lecture, 10/2015) suggested that we could reframe the model of "The Music Child" trapped within "The Condition Child" to a more modern conception, whereby the "condition" is any inner or outer obstacle in the way of becoming a more fully realized person. "In this way," says Aigen, "the model becomes a more universal one; a way of uniting all people rather than dividing us."

THE MUSICAL FORM ITSELF IS THE INTERVENTION

It is not as if there is an inherently non-musical experience which one is conveying through a particular musical form; rather, the musical form itself (idiom, rhythm, tension/resolution, melody, harmony, timbre, interval, scale, mode) is the intervention.

—*Dr. Kenneth Aigen (2001)*

The wording of Nordoff and Robbins's first book (reissued in 2005), *Therapy in Music for Handicapped Children*, immediately establishes the Nordoff-Robbins position. It is therapy in music—that is, the therapy is contained within, or intrinsic to, musical engagement. In other words, when a client is actively involved in music, therapy is occurring. Music therapy, in this sense, functions as does all artistic creation: through a process of discovery, often unpremeditated and unforeseeable, taking shape and unfolding moment by moment. We can have goals or certain preconceptions in mind, but if we are to stay true to the artistic process, we must be receptive to the direction, and possibly the benefits, of the work turning out differently than we had originally imagined. This view is sharply differentiated from that which would be implied by the reverse wording: music in therapy—that is, applying music as a device toward the purposes of some disparate clinical conception which may be partly or largely nonmusical. The precedent for all that was to become identified as the Nordoff-Robbins approach is clearly defined on the second page of the authors' introduction of *Therapy in Music for Handicapped Children* (2005):

Music therefore becomes a sphere of experience, a means of intercommunication and a basis for activity in which handicapped children can find freedom, in varying degrees, from the malfunctions that restrict their lives. As such, music possesses inherent capacities for effecting a uniquely significant contact with handicapped children and for providing an experiential ground for their engagement, their personality development, their integration—both individually and socially. To the extent to which music achieves this it becomes music therapy; in practice, the range of expression of music as an art, and the structural constitution of music as an artistic discipline, are directly involved. (p. 16)

The significance of this revolutionary declaration is astonishing considered within the social context of the early sixties, when Nordoff and Robbins began developing their initial ideas. Nordoff and Robbins embarked on their collaborative journey at the Sunfield Children's Homes for severely disabled children in England. The anthroposophical philosophy of

Sunfield, informed by the ideas of Rudolf Steiner, was extremely progressive for its time. A wide range of painting, music, movement, drama, and craft activities were consistently employed. Still, in subsequent writings, Clive Robbins described his extreme frustration at the seeming impossibility of penetrating the communication barriers of profound developmental disability and autism in children during his initial position there as a special education teacher.

Sunfield Homes notwithstanding, I would venture that expectations for severely disabled children in those days were rather limited, and that in most institutional settings, musical endeavors, if any, were of the bad sing-along, plastic maraca-shaking variety. These types of condescending, mind-numbing interventions are, woefully, all too common, even today. Even in more sophisticated circles, the degree to which music therapy functions predominantly according to the nature of art and music, as opposed to music taking a subordinate position to psychoanalytic, behavioral, medical, or recreational principles, is as controversial today as it was in the fifties and sixties when the field first began to establish itself.

I think Nordoff and Robbins were well aware of their essential voices as pioneers and leaders in this relatively nascent field. "Music is a universal language" is virtually a platitude, and an empty one at that, if music therapists favor other "clinical strategies," and utilize music in a relatively superficial manner. As Nordoff and Robbins (2005) pointed out, "What has yet to be more clearly recognized is the range of expression that is possible in this language. The variety of human expression that can be communicated through music is highly diversified and virtually unlimited. Because of this, music becomes vitally important as therapy for exceptional [handicapped] children" (p. 49).

WE ARE HERE TO WORK

Many ideas, attitudes and practices in the early case studies of Nordoff and Robbins can be derived from their fundamental ideas about the nature of work and its role in human functioning and development.

—Dr. Kenneth Aigen (1998)

Work necessitates consciousness of one's activity.
Work requires the selective inhibition of energy, affect, and impulse.
Work requires frustration tolerance and the delay of gratification.
Work is an expression of will.
Work requires care, concentration, and reverence.
The rewards of work build up over time.

The ability to engage in meaningful work is a necessary component of psychological health because it gives meaning to life.

The focus during this early Nordoff-Robbins collaboration consisted exclusively of work with children. Although many of the musical pieces developed by Nordoff and Robbins addressed issues inherently meaningful to the children, none of them are, in any way, condescending, either musically or thematically. They invoke a high degree of alertness, challenge, and involvement, and the work involved in mastering them leads to a sense of having really accomplished something. I participated in some of them as a student. In particular, the exquisitely intricate "hist-whist" stands out in my mind.

This full-length composition (based on an e.e. cummings Halloween-type poem for children) encompasses specific orchestrations for a group of children. During my training, I worked on it with my fellow students for the whole of a two-hour class and, personally, never achieved anything one could honestly describe as mastery (although to be fair to myself, I seem to remember trying to cover two parts). If this was music for handicapped children, the clients must have intuitively realized that, for once, someone (or "something" inherent in music) was taking them seriously, offering them an opportunity to rise to the occasion. Regarding this, it is noted:

> *The piece took three-and-a-half minutes to perform, but eight sessions, each an hour and fifteen minutes in length, were required to perfect it. This is where the therapy lay. Once weekly the "sextet" met and worked hard without pause, learning and practicing the piece, section by section. The children accepted the therapists' single-minded purposefulness in the same spirit; they shared their enthusiasm and gave themselves completely to the hard musical work the piece demanded. Observers of the sessions, who knew the children, were incredulous over their capacity to sustain this kind of complete concentration for over an hour. (Nordoff-Robbins 2005, Appendix II)*

INDEXING AND ASSESSMENT

Nordoff and Robbins meticulously documented their work and observations. This continues today with the practice of indexing (detailed session notes) and assessment using the N-R Scales.

Every session is filmed, and part of the Nordoff-Robbins therapist's day is devoted to reviewing the video and making detailed notes. This degree of veneration and devotion of time to the music therapy process is virtually unique to Nordoff-Robbins and often yields observations and insights of which the therapist was not cognizant during the session. Additionally, it provides a record of fruitful improvisations that might be otherwise forgotten by the next session but now can be developed.

Nordoff-Robbins also designed assessment scales such as: "Categories of Response," which outlines thirteen categories (with various subcategories) for evaluating a child's manner of participating in music (for example, Complete Rhythmic Freedom, Compulsive Beating, Evasive Beating, Responses by Singing, and Responses to Specific Musical Idioms), and the Relationship Scale, which assesses the client's willingness to enter into music with the therapist versus the level of resistance.

A review of contemporary music therapy literature reflects a diversity of assessment scales designed for work with children, but most of them evaluate behavioral tasks that are seemingly unrelated to the dynamic musical relationship that naturally occurs between client and therapist. To this day, the Nordoff-Robbins Scales remain in the minority of music-centered assessment instruments utilized in the field. (*The Individual Music-Centered Assessment Profile for Neurodevelopmental Disorders: A Clinical Manual* [2013], designed by noteworthy Nordoff-Robbins alumnus, John Carpente, is another.)

MUTUALITY

> *The efficacy of any course of music therapy is determined by the degree to which the therapist can fully insert his or her own being into the music and elicit a similar commitment on the part of the [client]. Once this is accomplished, all the variety of dynamic experience latent in the musical forms becomes accessible to the client—experiences not typically available to the [client] due to his or her pathology.*
>
> —*Dr. Kenneth Aigen (1996, p. 12)*

In understanding the origins of such a profound focus on music, we cannot underestimate the significance of Nordoff's background as a serious composer, university professor, and virtuoso pianist. This was not a man to play some insipid version of a children's song and leave it at that. The depth of Nordoff's commitment to putting his former career aside in order to investigate the possibilities of music therapy, coupled with Robbins's emancipation from the limitations of special education, and the sense of possibility and rejuvenation they felt is illustrated by passages such as this one:

The therapist feels reborn in his new musical therapeutic experiences and realizes the art of music as therapy will never cease to challenge him, never cease to require all his musical resources. As mediator of therapeutic music he assumes new, uplifting responsibilities. Out of his love for music he approaches handicapped children musically, feels them musically. Through his practical ability as a musician he works with them clinically. With his musical perceptiveness and musical intelligence he understands their responses artistically and humanly recognizes what they express. (Nordoff-Robbins 2005, p. 142)

THE ARCHETYPAL ASPECTS OF MUSIC

The archetypal aspects of music reach beyond the client's present self to elicit developmental potentials and assist in the integration of the personality.

—Dr. Alan Turry (1998)

From their very first project, at Herbert Geuter's suggestion (Sunfield's treatment team director), Nordoff and Robbins plunged in with a sense of passion and discovery. They believed that music carried primal forces that could be employed for clinical benefit. Spanish music was not the same as Middle Eastern music, and this was not the same as an English folk ballad. And lush harmonies played in the lower register of the piano were not the same as a simple melody played in the upper register. Each approach had its own dynamic qualities and could open up different clinical potentials.

One early example involved work with a hypertonic epileptic boy at Sunfield who could only take small, awkward steps and was unable to raise his arms above his shoulders. Dr. Geuter prescribed a specific movement—to take a big stride and at the same time thrust his arms outward, spreading them above his head. Nordoff (1998) described his musical "treatment":

He was to attempt to make this large free movement by his own efforts to a rhythm, one often found in Spanish music. . . . After seven months, having worked thrice weekly, he was able to perform it successfully. As a result all his movements became freer and the tensions that had hindered his mixing with others began to ease. His speech became less strained and gained in fluency. The strongly accented accompaniment in the Spanish idiom I used was an essential part of the treatment. (p. 27)

Nordoff and Robbins's belief in the transpersonal forces in the musical forms (modes, idioms from diverse parts of the world, use of complex harmonies, dissonance) reach for an inherent or universal disposition or potential within the client with which the archetype has affinity (Nordoff, 1998), as in this example:

> *One fact, however, emerged: dynamic, dissonant music does not necessarily excite or disturb psychotic children. . . . As I aimed to express the turbulence of their emotional lives in the music I improvised, it was often wild and dissonant. This experience appeared to be more significant than quiet, soothing music which might have been considered more suitable. (p. 41)*

The courage involved in resisting the dominant sentiment of the time cannot be overstated and is no less germane an issue today. However, at least when contemporary music therapists engage in methodological debates with other professionals or administrators, they have Nordoff-Robbins and those who followed in their path to substantiate the work. Nordoff and Robbins had only their own convictions, as they recounted:

> *The visits to Sonnenhof, Switzerland and Bingenheim, Germany were important because of the clarification of concepts our experiences there demanded. Both institutions placed great value on music in the lives of their children and in the discussions that took place we were seriously challenged to justify our use of music. Many workers found much of it too loud, too dissonant and too rhythmic. They were of the opinion that music for handicapped children should be soothing, rather soft, conventionally harmonious, and, if active, not stimulating. (Nordoff-Robbins 2005, p. 44)*

Music is not meant to be approached as some type of soporific musical participation that is more of a mild form of entertainment than music therapy. Music is not meant to be a subduing, conditioning factor in a client's life. In providing an alternative to such anemic applications, Nordoff and Robbins's (2005) resolute dedication to their vision can be pinpointed in this statement: "Music, we fervently believe, could be more than this" (p. 45).

CHANGES IN MUSICAL EXPRESSION ARE SEEN AS SIGNIFICANT CHANGES IN SELF

> *Musical expression is an expression of the self. Within the therapeutic relationship, we work toward musical experiences that will impact the core of each person. When a client's music is changing, he or she is changing. There is no differentiation between the two.*
>
> *—Dr. Alan Turry (1998)*

In Nordoff-Robbins music therapy there is license to express clinical goals in purely musical terms. Therapists must develop sharp sensitivity and awareness in detecting and responding to changes in a client's music, for example:

- improved vocal range or pitch
- stronger rhythmic groove
- increased flexibility and freedom
- greater ability to collaborate
- more confidence, inventiveness, or focus in playing

Identifying and supporting such musical progress requires a substantial musician. Right from the start, Nordoff and Robbins held us all up to the highest standard of clinical music, and I think many music therapists with lesser chops might be intimidated, justifiably so. As a guitarist beginning my training, I was certainly aware that it simply would not do for my musical resources to be confined to the rhythmic strumming with full, consonant chords and predictable tonal resolution to which many guitarists are habituated. I needed to cultivate a more highly developed sense of clinical presence and musical dexterity as I experimented with techniques that generated the tensions, dissonances, modal influences, use of intervals, diverse harmonies, idioms, and flexible rhythms that seemed true to the criterion set by Nordoff and Robbins (2005), as in this description:

> *All the compositional styles of the last seven centuries, all the folk music, the idioms, the elements of music, the very notes themselves—even the smallest expressive and structural components—become significant in countless, undreamed-of ways. The world of music opens anew, now disclosing an inner musical life of therapeutic potential. (p. 142)*

LIVING IN THE CREATIVE NOW

> *Both therapist and client are living as completely as possible in the music. When this occurs, one's entire physical, emotional and spiritual being is becoming manifest in the music and the music functions as an extension of the person*
>
> *—Dr. Kenneth Aigen (1996, p. 12)*

The *Creative Now* is a term coined by Clive Robbins. When we walk into a music therapy session, we have the known: memorized repertoire, forms, styles, techniques, chops, and approaches with which we've had experience; everything we've done before. Then we have the unknown:

the inspirations, intuitions, and improvisations yet to come. And in the middle of all that is this moment—the Now. All artists create from a place of no mind, said Eckhart Tolle (2004). The letting go of mental-emotional resistance to what is—to the now—becomes a portal into the *unmanifested*.

As therapists, we cannot stand back dispassionately and apply music like some sort of quasi-medical treatment and expect to facilitate a creative environment that has any heart. We enter a session in service to our clients. At the same time, in music we are united. Two or more people playing together generate one sound, one creation. The purpose of music therapy is to offer an opportunity to step outside of the restrictive boundaries imposed by society, pathology, and ego-isolation. Our objective is to enter into the all embracing, ever renewing, moment-to-moment world of music with our clients and help them to return with something new; maybe something they can use.

A NEW MORAL REALITY

> *As [the therapist] leads and follows the child into new regions of self-expression, into new discoveries of freedom, his joy is the child's joy, his fulfillment is the child's fulfillment. The relationship he has to the child's self-creating self through the creative effort of his music-making, gives his own musical nature—and with it the art of music—a new moral reality in the world*
>
> —*Nordoff and Robbins (2005, p. 144)*

Music in modern times has, to a great extent, been trivialized, marginalized, and characterized primarily as entertainment or relegated to the background. Pop music is a billion-dollar industry, classical concerts fill halls, jazz aficionados gather in dark clubs, folkies travel to festivals, wedding bands play endless parties. Music is used to create a desired atmosphere in films, television commercials, and shopping malls. Entire careers are devoted to criticizing it, analyzing it, and merchandizing it. Our lives are saturated with music, yet somehow it all seems so frivolous.

Legions of musicians continue to nurture the dream of becoming rich and famous. Nordoff, himself, was on sabbatical from his university to further his composing career in Europe when he was first introduced to the idea of music as therapy. Had his original intent worked out more to his satisfaction, I would venture that the Nordoff-Robbins partnership would never have happened. It was frustration—Nordoff's with the music profession and Robbins's with the special education system—that led to the need to look beyond the way things were and create something different.

Perhaps it is a cliché or a generalization to say that the most potent music arises out of a mood of social or personal oppression, but I still think it is basically true. Music may be promoted as an entertainment and star-making business to serve the purposes of a capitalist culture, but this is not its reality. In music, we are able to transcend the loneliness, fear, and constraint inherent in the experience of being human. As Nordoff and Robbins noted, within handicapped children live some of the deepest needs of humanity, and this is why music can become so important in their lives. But as music therapists, we are not simply providers. In participating in music that has been restored to a context more worthy of its essence, we are all renewed. This intensely humanistic, even spiritual, perspective lives at the heart of the Nordoff-Robbins approach.

I have come to many of my views about music therapy largely through the example of Nordoff and Robbins. This is certainly not to suggest that my opinions represent a consensus among Nordoff-Robbins therapists or that there even is one. It is, in fact, its diversity, encouraging dialogue, and debate that makes the Nordoff-Robbins approach so vital fifty years after the initial publication of their first book, *Therapy in Music for Handicapped Children* (first published in 1971). Since then, many additional brilliant insights, elucidations, and interpretations were set to paper by Nordoff and Robbins, Clive and Carol Robbins, Clive by himself, the many notable Nordoff-Robbins–trained clinicians, and other kindred spirits. But Nordoff and Robbins created the paradigm that, like any great work of art, responded to the needs of its time as much as it illuminates the future.

THOMAS: BEING IN MUSIC

My work with Thomas was, perhaps, my greatest training ground in strengthening my conviction and skill in a music-centered approach. It occurred while I was engaged in post-master's certification training at the New York University Nordoff-Robbins Center for Music Therapy, commencing October 2000 and concluding June 2002. The personnel in the session included myself and co-therapist center director Dr. Alan Turry, who was my training supervisor. The Nordoff-Robbins Center videotapes every moment of every session. Volunteers made up of NYU students and other interested people film from a hidden booth, enabling the video to follow the action, employing close-ups, wide shots, and other film techniques. This not only enables the clinician to closely review the work later, but also to edit together important moments, creating a compelling longitudinal video document.

Because of the richness of the work and accompanying video, I have presented my Thomas case study at numerous venues: conferences, seminars, lectures for the public, and university classes. I also documented his case in the journal, *Music Therapy Perspectives* (Soshensky, 2005). In addition to my own presentations, Clive Robbins included the study in his international lecture circuit. I think Clive appreciated it so much because Thomas is adorable and charismatic and made dramatic progress over the course of the study but mostly because I focused on guitar as a primary instrument during the training. Clive told me he wanted to illustrate the adaptability of the Nordoff-Robbins approach beyond the original piano-based model as established by Paul Nordoff. I am truly honored and humbled to have been afforded the opportunity to fulfill that role for him.

Clive Robbins was a rare individual—inspiring, profound, and charismatic in a way that few people are. Yet when he spoke to you, he had this totally focused presence as if, at that moment, you were the most important person in the world to him. And you were. The lessons I learned from him, Dr. Turry, and everyone at the Nordoff-Robbins Center are unparalleled in my growth as a music therapist. Although I was an accomplished musician and a somewhat experienced therapist when I started the training, my heightened sensitivity and sophistication in listening musically and working in the creative now, in playing with compositional awareness and intention, in making the client's responses vital to the ongoing musical process—these were not remotely as developed going in as going out. The reader will notice the attention to musical detail in keeping with Nordoff-Robbins's deeply music-centered convictions.

Here's Thomas

Thomas was a two-and-a-half-year-old boy who had been diagnosed with pervasive developmental disorder and motor planning problems (the diagnosis was changed to autism when Thomas got older). Thomas had not developed any language nor had he vocalized much at all beyond crying. He was highly anxious and could not settle down to take naps or sleep peacefully through the night. He had poorly developed body awareness and did not use his hands purposefully to manipulate objects such as eating utensils, door knobs, or toys. As he began to walk, he seemed not to know where he was in space, and his mother reported that, in spite of normal vision, he was literally walking into walls. Social interaction was essentially nonexistent other than nervously clinging to his mother. He could not tolerate crowds, ignored his four-year-old brother, and did not engage in play.

On my first day as a Nordoff-Robbins therapist-in-training, I strove to use all my compositional and empathic skills as I improvised a gentle, folk-ballad-style song, with the only lyric, "Here's Thomas." Despite his apparent tentativeness, Thomas seemed to respond positively to music during his first session. He swayed from side to side, made intermittent eye-contact, and smiled several times, revealing glimpses of an engaging and attractive personality. Otherwise, his facial expression remained flat, and he often seemed to focus off into the distance or up toward the ceiling. He appeared musically sensitive, however, as evidenced by alert glances and changes in swaying motion in response to variations in harmony and rhythm. He didn't seem to like it when I slowed the tempo too much or stopped playing, as he turned anxiously to his mother (who attended the first seven sessions) until the music started again, whereupon he would recommence his swaying.

Thomas grasped several small instruments that we offered him in the first few sessions, such as shaker eggs and small bells, but he held them for only a moment before dropping them, and he didn't utilize them in any musical manner. He showed no interest in any other instruments in the room and moved to the door several times within the half-hour session. Although he didn't appear overly distressed, when his attention was not fully engaged, his thoughts seemed to turn to leaving. Based on the first few sessions which proceeded in this manner, along with information provided by his mother, I formulated the following goals for Thomas:

- To tolerate a full session without attempting to withdraw
- To develop ability to initiate and sustain musical interaction
- To enjoy music as a meaningful form of play and fun
- To develop a sense of trust and cooperative interaction with therapists
- To develop use of voice
- To utilize instruments with musical purpose and intent
- To increase body awareness through playing instruments and movement to music
- To freely express needs/preferences and feelings within our session

Falling Asleep

During the third session, Thomas moved freely about the room and interacted comfortably with Alan and me. He would not engage musically, however, and after about fifteen minutes he became lethargic and sat down in a plastic, child-size cube chair. I tried some energetic music, but in spite of this, he fell into a deep sleep. We did not end the session, however, but transferred the sleeping Thomas from the chair to Alan's lap. This decision was partially influenced by the account of Herr G. that I had recently read in Gary Ansdell's book *Music for Life* (1995). It describes a man who recovered fully from a supposedly hopeless coma and later reported that not only was he aware of the music therapist singing to him while in his coma, but he also credited it with helping him to find his way back to consciousness. So with the assumption that sleep was no barrier to music, I moved in quite close with my guitar and improvised a bass note melody in A minor while singing in unison. I thought the full, earthy vibrations of the bass might be more easily "felt" in his sleep state, and the deep minor melody sounded reverent—a bit like a Gregorian chant. Thomas's mother was moved to weeping as she witnessed the relaxed state of her little boy who could not sleep. Thomas left the session in his stroller sound asleep, and his mother reported that his sleep patterns at home began to improve following this session.

Awakening

A few weeks later, Thomas arrived for his session having fallen asleep in his stroller on the way to the Center. Clearly, this was a little boy who was learning to take naps! This time, however, I decided to wake him, so I asked his mother to move him gently while I sang and played a rubato melody, primarily in a Dorian mode rooted in D. I just happened to realize later that I played in the Dorian mode. I didn't make a conscious decision about that at the time. I had tuned my guitar's low E on the sixth string down to a D, creating full modal sound with the root-fifth-octave (D-A-D) organum in the bass strings. Although I did this primarily to provide an encompassing and supportive musical environment into which Thomas would awaken, it is notable that throughout history, specific attributes have been ascribed to the modes. Socrates believed that the Dorian mode "emboldens warriors and helps them to accept and cope with setbacks" (James, 1993, p. 57).

Thomas did, indeed, seem emboldened and encouraged by this music. As he became more alert, I offered the chimes to him, and, to my surprise, he reached out and began to play them. This was the first time he had actively participated in music. As in the previous example, I was positioned very close to Thomas as we sat on the floor together creating an intimate circle of sound. The pulse remained relaxed, yet the sound of the modal guitar and the chimes swelling and receding together created a moving experience. In the video, we can see Thomas turn to his mother several times with an expression that seemed to say: "What is this?" communicating an awakening awareness of our musical relationship that was stirring within him.

Thomas Finds His Voice

After that, Thomas began showing greater trust and enjoyment, and beginning with the eighth session, he started coming into the music room without his mother. Chime playing was still the only active playing in which he was willing to engage and, although it initially seemed significant, it soon became difficult to discern whether he was engaging musically or lost in self-absorption. As we experimented with other ways to involve him, a musical theme developed with an energetic Celtic influence, like an Irish jig, during which Alan supported Thomas in a rhythmic jumping dance movement on a large drum. Thomas seemed to love this, and soon a second section developed, wherein Thomas held his hands up above his head, which meant he wanted Alan to lift him up and move him around in a flying motion. During this, I switched to a freer, less pulse-driven theme in 3/4 time in a minor key.

The piece was revisited numerous times and began to evolve. During a particularly active session in the fifth month of therapy, Thomas was jumping enthusiastically and smiling joyfully. I switched from the Celtic feel to more of a straight 4/4 "country/rock" feel, improvising freely over the solid rhythm of Thomas's assisted drum-jumping. I used no chordal accompaniment, allowing the driving rock-style, single-string, and two-string lines, along with the pounding drum, to define the character of the piece.

This invigorating music offered a striking contrast to the mellow waltz of the "flying" section. Alan lifted Thomas up as he had done many times previously. This time, however, Thomas let out a melodic "ooo" vocal sound. It was the first time he had used his voice! I immediately stood up with my guitar and came up to him, continuing the music face-to-face, in order to acknowledge and enhance this momentous breakthrough. I didn't display my elation, however, because this was his moment, not mine. I simply reflected his tone and then initiated some of my own to see if he would respond to me as we moved around the room. He did, but only on the vowel sounds, "ooo" and "ahh."

The drum-jumping and flying music continued for quite a while, alternating from jumping to flying, based on Thomas's cues, and the extensive vocal interplay continued throughout the remainder of the session. Following this session, Thomas's mother reported dramatic progress with his speech therapist, including increased vocalizations (with occasional singing) and the beginning of word use at home.

> *The world is all gates, all opportunities, strings of tension waiting to be struck.*
>
> —*Emerson (2010)*

Eventually, Thomas began to engage in brief moments of playing on melodic instruments, such as a small xylophone. Although using his hands and interacting musically was meaningful, his involvement was fleeting and unpredictable. I still often gravitated toward full, six-string, folk-influenced strums typical of acoustic guitar. The music could be energetic or calm, but was generally rhythmic and consonant sounding. I hoped that Thomas would want to add a musical part on top of these secure accompaniment patterns, but this approach met with little success. Instances of Thomas's early melodic instrument playing were mostly in response to unstable music such as:

- "bluesy" bent notes slurred into micro-tones
- sudden pauses
- dissonant harmonies
- unresolved melodic lines
- surprising shifts in dynamics, rhythm, or harmony

This music seemed to capture his attention and call for his participation to help it find some organization and rest. Nordoff supported this kind of approach in contrast to the simple melodies often thought of as children's music, asserting: "When we're improvising for a child, we can bring in tension, release it, bring it in, deepen it, intensify it. Use tones that have an urgency to go somewhere" (Robbins & Robbins, 1998, p. 123). Clive (personal communication, May 24, 2002) also encouraged this, telling me the ability "to move the music, not just have it be a comfortable thing, is the essence of our work."

Accepting the Emotional-Expressive Reality and Meeting It Musically

It took me a while to learn this lesson. I began the twenty-third session, in the eighth month of therapy by, once again, strumming full chords and singing a melodic vocal line, trying to inspire Thomas to join me by playing beautiful tones on a C-diatonic metalophone that I had placed in front of him. One thing he shortly discovered about this particular metalophone was that even though its tone bars were fastened on one side, they were not fastened on the other. This enabled him to pick up one side of the bar and let it drop with a metallic "clang." For Thomas, this seemed more appealing than playing with a mallet, and he paid little attention to me or my music. Applying one of the most fundamental principles in Nordoff-Robbins music therapy, I decided to accept what he was doing "as an emotional-expressive reality in the situation and meet it musically" (Nordoff & Robbins, 1977, p. 27). I abandoned the idea of trying to encourage pleasant sounding music and began to play chords containing dissonant intervals such as flat-seven, sharp-nine, tritone, flat-nine. Every time he dropped a bar, I hit a dissonant chord with a harsh attack, reflecting the sound of the falling metal bars.

We proceeded in this manner and, at one point, I played a dissonant chord five times in a rapid sixteenth note rhythm. I thought Alan responded to this as a funk reference, as he let out a James Brown–like "Ow!" Although he later said he wasn't thinking that at all, funk music frequently utilizes dissonant intervals but, certainly, its most defining feature is its relentless, syncopated rhythm. As I added a "funky" strum to the dissonant chords, Thomas stopped what he was doing, raised his head, and looked around with an expression that clearly indicated his recognition of this new music. With a little smile on his face, he picked up a mallet and began to play in tempo with the guitar.

As we continued, there were times when Thomas began to lose contact with the music or went back to dropping bars. The contrast between the powerful groove implicit in the funk style and Thomas's wavering time and inconsistent playing represented a major turning point for me. I learned how to not be a "slave to the rhythm" (apologies to Grace Jones). As Turry later commented, "I think you broke out of a certain habitual way that people use guitar where the tempo stays in one place so you can then sing above it" (personal communication, May 24, 2002). Guitarists can become conditioned to this type of approach, but in this case I needed to be responsive to Thomas's rhythmic deviations if I was to maintain contact with him. This required me to diverge from a strict "funk" interpretation by slowing down at times, leaving space as necessary, and returning to the music of dropping bars for a bit. Yet even when his rhythm faltered, the subliminal momentum that the funk idiom established seemed to provide an impetus that impelled Thomas forward and unified our music. By allowing for this malleability with my time and music, I kept Thomas engaged and successfully used the funk idiom for the most interactive and sustained playing he had yet achieved.

Inner Balance

By the last session of Thomas's first year of music therapy before a summer break, he had played drums, as well as other melodic instruments, and piano. A sense of shared responsibility began to develop in our improvisations as he acted with more initiative and generated more musical ideas. During this final session of the year, Thomas played a G pentatonic xylimba while I accompanied without a fixed pulse, using lightly picked major and minor thirds, single string melody, and moments of silence as I responded to Thomas's reflective playing, pauses, and glissandi. Nordoff described thirds as positive statements of inner balance. Perhaps this music offered a few moments of serenity and calm coactivity which Thomas may have seldom experienced.

Olé: The Spanish Idiom

After a two-month break for the summer, we began our second year of therapy. Thomas was far more lively and extroverted, moving around the room freely and playing drums, cymbal, piano, and other melodic instruments. His playing, although still sporadic, displayed increased organization. He also vocalized loudly with elongated, musical phrasing, often on the word, "No!" Rather than being an objection to anything in particular, it seemed more to reflect Thomas's awakening sense of personal power and his increasing artistic license for self-expression in music.

In trying to find the right music to compliment his energy, I was drawn to a Phrygian mode in a Spanish Flamenco style. This music is usually considered to have a strong rhythmic component, but it also has a unique way of holding and releasing tension. Turry explains:

> *The harmonic cadences can be more subtle than in rock or jazz—they can be extended and often times rubato playing serves to stretch out the resolution of phrases. There is less a feeling of being locked in a groove by a steady tempo and more of a feeling of constantly renewed rhythmic drive. (Cited in Wagner, 1999, p. 9)*

This provided containment without confinement in response to Thomas's free playing, singing, and varied activity in the room. It allowed us to establish a forceful rhythm, then quickly shift to quiet rubato playing, rapidly strummed chords, even charged silence, then back into a compelling pulse. Because of the idiom's adaptability, Thomas's mercurial participation did not feel disjointed. He vocalized, offered musical accents, completed unresolved phrases on a drum or a cymbal, and within the embrace of Spanish music, his musical impulses formed the basis for various movements in a coherent whole.

Composition and Adaption

Midway through the second year, a pivotal song developed. "Let's Go!," as it became known, had a bouncy feel, with Latin and Caribbean influences. With a little assistance from Alan, Thomas quickly picked up on the idea of the drumbeat landing on the first downbeat of the two-bar chorus. This was not planned, but once it took shape, we were able to expand on the concept. I held the V chord while singing, "Let's . . ." for an extended period until Thomas hit the decisive drumbeat on "Go!" which led us to the beginning of the progression. Thomas seemed to derive great joy from this discovery of a specific part to play and in having such an important role in controlling the flow of the music. "Let's Go!" originally had another section, but this became extraneous as we played the two-bar chorus countless times per session. Because of the interaction, fun, and variation involved in the perpetual cycle of tension/resolution, it never became boring. "Let's Go!" established itself as a very important clinical theme, lasting many months, virtually never failing to arouse Thomas's interest and inspire his involvement when his attention would wane.

As the piece evolved, I began to transform the V chord, a D7, to an E♭ diminished chord, simply by raising the D in the bass one-half step to an E♭. This one-note alteration in the harmony greatly increased the suspense of the fermata as I sang, "Let's . . ." Nordoff (cited in Robbins & Robbins, 1998) called the diminished chord "one of the most powerful chords in music" and one "you can really say is a chord of conflict" (p. 47). Sometimes, I moved back and forth between the D7 chord and the diminished, holding off the resolving beat indefinitely, continuously escalating the climatic energy. During this music Thomas jumped with exhilaration and looked at me expectantly, hitting the cymbal to accentuate the tension until his drumbeat on the snare brought us back to "Go!" This process noticeably strengthened our musical relationship, as well as Thomas's confidence and self-awareness.

Arrangement and Rehearsal

Thomas's parents informed me that, although he was achieving important milestones, he was unable to sustain attention for long at home or at his preschool. For example, they said, he would occasionally sit down to draw, but he would typically make a line or two and then abandon the project. Likewise, his music still gave the impression of being a series of fragmented sections that could be discontinued at any time. Consequently, about three quarters of the way into our second year, a new clinical goal emerged:

- To further the experience of music as an aesthetically meaningful whole, sustained to a sense of completion

I introduced "Simon's Bells," a composition by Dr. Suzanne Sorel (1999). This flowing ballad utilizes a simple five-note ascending and descending major scale that is easy to play, but is supported by a beautiful harmonic accompaniment, providing richness, movement, and tension. Playing an arranged melody was well beyond what Thomas had done so far, but I hoped he would come to see the piece as indivisible, finding fulfillment in seeing it through to its conclusion.

A metalophone was set up with the five-note do-re-me-fa-so scale, leaving space between each bar to make it easier for Thomas to strike the tones precisely using a mallet. We worked with "Simon's Bells" over several sessions, playing it numerous times. Various methods were used in helping Thomas to master the piece. While I sang and played the song, Alan demonstrated Thomas's part, assisted him hand-over-hand, pointed to the tone bars he needed to play, and covered all the bars except the one he needed to play.

It was certainly a more directed process than the improvisations we had done previously, but instead of resisting or ignoring us, as he surely would have in the past, Thomas accepted the challenge. He learned his part, playing the tones mindfully, in the correct order and in time with the harmonic movement. He had some trouble with the descending section, but he made a concerted effort, seeming to appreciate the aesthetics of the music and the piece as a whole. By discovering the intrinsic reward in realizing the composition, he achieved new levels of organization, focused attention, and collaboration.

Outcomes

As we approached the end of Thomas's second year of music therapy, he had come to a point where he was able to thrive in the creative environment. He was four and a half years old, and his parents reported gains in many important areas:

- He slept normally.
- He was far more physically coordinated.
- He used his hands for activities and skills appropriate to his age.
- He had friends and sang with groups in school.
- His attention and focus was much improved.
- He played with his brother.
- His parents were able to read him stories.
- He tolerated crowds, such as parties and public events.
- His parents took him to the circus, which his father described as "a big thing."
- He understood and appreciated humor.
- His verbal communication improved.

Look for the music on all things, and life will be a symphony of joy.

—Stravinsky (1961)

Perhaps the most striking change in Thomas was his sense of fun. When he first arrived for music therapy, his affect was flat most of the time. He didn't know how to play. During our final session together,

Thomas jumped with excitement, smiled brightly, with direct eye contact, and radiated a vitality that was barely present earlier in the course of music therapy. As he filled in the key lyrics of our last good-bye song, the words were not always fully articulated, but his joy and enthusiasm expressed more than his language.

I had come to the end of my training, but Thomas continued at the Nordoff-Robbins Center for many years with other therapists, mostly in groups, to continue building on his substantial growth in social interaction, focus, and communication. My work with Thomas and other clients at the Nordoff-Robbins Center immeasurably enhanced my conviction that music approached as a creative art, with all its mystery and wild abandon, could still be navigated as a dynamic and effective form of therapy.

As of this writing, Thomas is twenty-two years old. He is happy, creative, and fully verbal. Although I've never had a reunion with him, I have spoken to his mother and she credits music therapy as being the bridge to all these essential life skills. If one reflects on the differing life paths of a verbal and socially capable person versus a nonverbal, socially disconnected person, the momentousness of Thomas's breakthroughs are apparent. Whether or not he would have eventually made progress in another way, without music therapy, is academic. The fact is, it was his journey through music that led him out of isolation, and I am profoundly grateful to have been a fellow traveler.

II

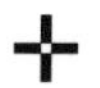

THE MUSIC THERAPY STUDIO: FRAMEWORK

5

Instruction and Practice

PRACTICE, PRACTICE, PRACTICE. THEN FORGET ALL THAT AND JUST WAIL

The above subtitle, a paraphrasing of a statement attributed to jazz great Charlie Parker (Pugatch, 2006), highlights the idea that the technical aspect of music is not the same as the actual experience of making music. Instruction and practice in music therapy are different from instruction and practice in a traditional lesson or school. A music therapist is a guide and a partner in exploring the musical landscape, but we are not the authoritarian, all-knowing expert professor or master teacher. My way of thinking about it is more in line with the words of writer/poet, Kahlil Gibran (2009):

> *The teacher who walks in the shadow of the temple, among his followers, gives not of his wisdom but rather of his faith and his lovingness. If he is indeed wise he does not bid you enter the house of his wisdom, but rather leads you to the threshold of your own mind. For the vision of one man lends not its wings to another man.*

I don't focus on the technical side of music at all, such as accurate pitch in singing, hitting the right notes, or rhythms in playing. I emphasize the communicative, expressive, relationship building qualities of music. In any case, over time, clients naturally improve through doing. Barbara Crowe (2004) pointed out that music therapy can develop ego strength and improved self-concept through successful playing experiences and accomplishments that are obvious to the client. No external feedback is necessary. If a therapist wants to acknowledge or compliment something, fine, but it might be best to avoid constant praise. The ubiquitous "Good job!" is overused with special needs children (and even adults), commonly proclaimed at the slightest achievement that would go unnoticed in a typical person. Even a major accomplishment might have less meaning lost in an endless sea of "Good jobs!"

Even though I don't push for the repetition and refining of a piece the way a teacher might, there is still value to this natural activity of music. Developing and perfecting repertoire can strengthen essential personal attributes that may generalize outside of music:

- Patience
- Persistence
- Discipline
- Frustration tolerance
- Goal achievement
- Collaboration
- Humility
- Awareness of growth

When should a music therapist push for a specific musical result? When should he or she "go with the flow"? When might preparing for community or public expression be appropriate? One way to know might be the expressed wish of the client. Or, if the therapist is trying to push a client to get something correct and he or she is becoming overwhelmed, frustrated, or irritated, it might be best to back off. We are leader as well as follower seeking a shared agenda, one goal.

> *You've got to be half inviting and half directing; a mixture of the two, so that your direction at the same time is an invitation*
>
> *—Clive Robbins (in Aigen, 1996, p. 18)*

SUSANNAH: FACING THE CHALLENGES OF AUTISM

Susannah is a woman in her 30s who describes herself as living with high-functioning autism. She has a passion for singing, but previously had few opportunities to do it. In the studio, we find songs she likes, particularly oldies and songs from Broadway musicals. We find the right key for her. We build her repertoire and we practice. Sometimes she has asked to run vocal scale exercises like a traditional singing lesson.

We have found supportive, low-pressure places for her to perform her music. She finds great enjoyment and satisfaction in this. When we practice, I might give her feedback on pitch or interpretation or maybe suggest she put a little more feeling or an expressive movement into her song. It could be very much like a rehearsal. We have performed several times now, and each time Susannah seemed a little more relaxed. As we were performing or rehearsing, a smile, a happy giggle, some rhythmic body movement, came a little more freely.

Susannah has refused to allow autism to cast her in the role simply of a receiver of services. She has empowered herself to live as full a life as possible. She works and lives independently and has chosen to access music therapy to continue growing and learning to face the challenges of autism. Susannah has to work harder than most to fit in. Table 5.1 lists some things Susannah has identified about how autism affects her life and how Music Therapy helps.

Table 5.1.

Challenges of Autism	*In Music Therapy*
Primarily a visual learner; slow at auditory processing	Improved auditory processing through practicing and learning through music.
Struggles with anxiety and panic attacks	Music helps to relieve stress. While in music, one can let go of problems, concerns, and fears.
Worries a lot about the future	Music helps to focus on the present; performing can help one to feel good about oneself, and to feel one is achieving a goal.
Rigidity in thinking	Increased comfort with flexibility and making choices; for example, songs to keep in repertoire or songs to drop, what key is best, and trying new things such as playing percussion.
Social difficulties	Opportunities to relate socially through music; possible to perform with and for others.
Repetitive thoughts; can become fixated on thoughts or ideas	Rehearsing a song numerous times is normal in music. Adding improvements or variations allows for flexibility before moving on to another song after a while. Songs can frame thoughts and feelings in a context outside of oneself.
Literal thinking, rigidity of affect and body, struggles to understand other peoples' sense of humor	Music helps with lightheartedness and sense of fun loosening of affect, release of body tension through rhythm and movement to music.
Difficulty concentrating on sounds to be focused on and filtering out other sounds in the environment (e.g., cars going by, people talking outside the room)	Able to focus on music during session to the exclusion of background sounds.

Susannah's experience reveals the distinction between cognitively/linguistically oriented therapy and therapy through musical experience. Ethnomusicology professor Michael Bakan (2018) points out:

> *Because we live in a linguo-centric society, where language is so referential, certain words mean certain things, the connotations of the way you use a word, the gestures you make when you utter something, are so deeply coded and so open for being misinterpreted or manipulated if you don't do it right, that if you are set up differently neuro-cognitively (i.e., autistic), that can generate a lot of anxiety. Whereas the kinds of environments in which music is made are more sympathetic to a more neuro-diverse theater of operation in which people can find meaningful ways in which to interact and communicate.*

BIONEURO MUSIC THERAPY

The activation of virtually the entirety of the neural network involved in music-making may produce cross-modal effects in other behavioral or cognitive operations. Neuroplasticity, the capacity of the brain to continually adapt, modify (and repair or compensate in the case of damage) its structural and functional organization in response to experience, may partially explain the sensorimotor, emotional, and cognitive shifts that can be associated with music. It was once thought that the adult brain retained minimal plasticity, but recent evidence has demonstrated that structural changes occur in the brain throughout life, including the generation of new neurons and other brain cells and connections between and among neurons. It is important to note that neuroplasticity is influenced by the behaviors an individual engages in, as well as the environment in which an individual lives, works, or plays (Gage, 2004). This is a clear rationale for music therapy with its capacity to provide the neurologically stimulating effects of music listening, improvisation, performance, and composition which are spread throughout the brain and bio-neurological system (Levitan, 2006). The following may help to offer a basic understanding.

Neurological Influences of Playing Music

- **Increased Activity in the Corpus Callosum**—the bridge between the two hemispheres allowing messages to get across the brain faster and through more diverse routes
- **Improved Executive Function**—related to planning, attention to detail, and simultaneous analysis and integration of both cognitive and emotional aspects

- **Enhanced Emotional Processing**—through activation of the amygdala, hypothalamus, hippocampus, and nucleus accumbent (Levitan, 2006)

Biochemical Responses to Playing Music

- **Release of Oxytocin**—neurohormone related to positive social encounters, leading to increased trust, more eye contact, improved facial memory, increased generosity, and greater empathy
- **Increased Dopamine and Serotonin**—neurotransmitters related to positive mood and well-being
- **Decreased Stress Response**—decreased stress reaction hormones, lowered blood pressure and heart rate, inhibited negative emotional reactions

Table 5.2.

Music Skill	*Brain Area and Function*
Aesthetic/Artistic Expression, Composing, Collaboration, Awareness of Rhythm	**Prefrontal Cortex** involved with cognitive behavior, personality expression, decision-making, social behavior
Emotional Expression and Response	**Nucleus Accumbens, Amygdala, Hypothalmus** assessing and regulating emotion
Listening, Sensory Perception of Sound	**Auditory Cortex** processing of sound
Triggering of Memories Retaining of Music	**Hippocampus** processing learning and memory
Spatial Awareness, Touch, Body, Hands Feet, Fingers in Relation to Instrument	**Parietal Lobe** processing sensory information re: the location of body parts, interpreting visual info, processing language
Monitoring Hands, Reading Lyrics, Sheet Music	**Visual Cortex** processing visual info
Movement, Vocal Production, Swaying, Tapping, Using Motor Cortex, Hands and Feet for Instrument Playing	**Cerebellum** coordinating voluntary movement, maintain posture

WE ALL LEARN FROM EACH OTHER

A jazz pianist, a member of one of my groups, once commented on the role of the leader by reflecting that very early in his musical career, he deeply admired the great instrumental virtuosos. It was only much

> *later that he grew to understand that the truly great jazz musicians were those who knew how to augment the sound of others, how to be quiet, how to enhance the functioning of the entire ensemble.*
>
> —*Irvin Yalom (1995, p. 110)*

Renowned existential psychotherapist Irvin Yalom (1995) makes the point that, as practitioners, we are not trying to teach or be in charge as much as we are trying to help our clients become aware of their own potential. Yalom called client and therapist "fellow travelers" in therapy. We are all human beings dealing with the essential problems of existence, and we need to work cooperatively to solve them. We all learn from each other. The therapist is a teacher for the client. The client is a teacher for the therapist. One client is a teacher to another. In music therapy, we're not teaching or learning how to be better musicians. Although there is almost always improvement, it is a secondary consideration. We are learning to be happier, more functional human beings. Clients don't have to know it all or be perfectly healthy in order to be helpful to others. Dr. Yalom (2009) referred to the words of Nietzsche: "Some cannot loosen their own chains yet can nonetheless redeem their friends." Being of service to another is, perhaps, the most healing of all experiences.

"My clients are my greatest teachers" is a phrase I have heard numerous times since my student days at NYU. I believe it, but let's consider what it means. Hopefully, we learn how to be better music therapists, the more experience we have. But looking at the issue more deeply, Yalom (2009) referred to Carl Jung's belief about the increased efficacy of the wounded healer. Jung claimed that therapy worked best when the patient brought the perfect salve for the therapist's wound and that if the therapist doesn't change then the patient doesn't either. Perhaps if the therapist is willing to be open to his or her own vulnerability or essential humanness, there might be a greater capacity to engage more deeply and personally in the creative relationship. There are so many clients who have inspired me, whose being and lessons will stay in my mind and heart for my whole life. They're not people who tried to teach me something. They just did so through their spirit and our connection. I have learned numerous life lessons in the course of working with my clients:

- Don't take it personally.
- Accept people the way they are.
- Never give up on anyone.
- Always look for something good.
- People's courage can be enormous.
- Everyone wants to relate and be involved.

- Anyone can grow and change for the better.
- Everyone has gifts.

JAMES: BROKEN BRAIN

I've learned all these lessons in numerous ways from everyone with whom I've worked. Many have achieved amazing outcomes, but perhaps none more surprising and touching than James, a seemingly completely disconnected nonentity in a residential facility. Virtually everyone had given up on James long ago, but, amazingly, through music he became a well-integrated and appreciated member of his therapeutic community.

Don't Take It Personally

James was a 67-year-old man living in a long-term care facility dedicated primarily to the treatment of brain injury patients. He'd been in custodial care for his entire adult life due to chronic undifferentiated schizophrenia that emerged in adolescence, which was further complicated by a subsequent brain injury. Any family had long since disappeared from his life. James wandered around the facility in a slow, unassuming, and seemingly random way, occasionally sitting down somewhere. Usually, he sat by himself. Occasionally, he sat down briefly in a music group, seeming to be in a completely isolated and oblivious state, before getting up and moving on again.

I tried to engage James a few times, and he ignored me. I wasn't bothered or surprised by this, since James never spoke nor did he participate in anything or engage in any form of social interaction. Over the course of my career, there have been many more dramatic incidents and more difficult clients that necessitated that I not "take it personally," much more so than this gentle, vulnerable soul who appeared to be ignoring me. Nobody, neither staff nor any of the other patients, even tried to relate to James. His nurses helped him to dress, gave him his meals, and helped him to bed. In between, he wandered around. That was his day-to-day existence. If I thought of my needs over his and wanted to make my life a little easier, I would have written him off as had everyone else. And that almost happened.

Accept People the Way They Are

I noticed that James was coming to music groups more regularly. As usual, he would just sit down without participating, but his attendance became too frequent to be random. He seemed to like being there. He would show up at some point during the group, sit down, and often stay until the end, sometimes even after everyone else left, while my partner Peter and I were packing up our equipment cart in preparation to move it down the hall to the storage room.

I simply accepted James's presence. Sometimes I placed a drum in front of him, just in case. He never played it, and I didn't try to encourage him to do anything, incorrectly thinking, based on my few perfunctory attempts at connecting, that it would be fruitless. I thought welcoming him was good enough.

Never Give Up on Anyone

So, for what would happen next, I can take no credit. It was my partner Peter an extraordinarily sensitive, caring, and genuine soul, who one day, as we were packing up, asked James to hand him the drum that had been placed in front of him. James ignored Peter, so Peter repeated his request, eventually going right up to James, looking him in the eye, and asking him again in a warm, friendly way. James handed Peter the drum. This went on for a few weeks, with James gradually helping us more and more, eventually actually getting up to help pack up the cart. This was an amazing development in and of itself, until one day Peter asked James, "Do you want to push the cart to the storage room?" Although James never spoke, he did, on occasion, make little guttural sounds, and he said a quiet, raspy "eh," that sounded like assent to us. And it was, because James started pushing.

The corridor that we needed to travel en route from the music area to the storage room went past the administrative offices. As James was slowly pushing the cart, a secretary came out of the office with some papers, witnessed what was happening, and just about dropped whatever she was carrying. She stared for a moment and then ran back into the office, shortly coming out again with a few other administrative personnel, including the CEO. Then some more people noticed the scene and lined the corridor, staring in wide-eyed awe as if they were watching Nureyev dance "Swan Lake." Quite simply, anyone who knew James did not think he was capable of this level of human contact and participation.

Always Look for Something Good

After this revelation, James became something of a regular equipment assistant and, also, when we would offer him a drum in the music group, he would accept it, sometimes tapping lightly along to the music. The facility also offered biweekly writing sessions facilitated by a brilliant and intense local poet named Carolyn. One day I saw James in there writing. I didn't know he could write, so I stopped in to see what he was doing, and what I saw was a free-association stream of consciousness without any punctuation in large, shaky handwriting. Maybe most people would pay it little mind, other than the fact that he was doing something, and by now people were starting to accept his increased activity. But I noticed some themes in his poetic, Joycean flow of words. I like that kind of writing, having done a fair amount of it myself, and it made sense to me.

James continued coming to music groups, playing a little, staying until the end, and helping to pack up. A few other residents also began helping us pack up, so now we had our "road crew," of which James was part. He also continued to attend the poetry group on occasion, and I would often stop by to say hello and to see what he was writing. One day I looked at his paper and saw the usual flow of James's inner monologue, but one section stood out for me. It seemed to be saying something about his condition. I extracted it, writing it on a separate paper in stanza form, and showed it to James. I was very enthusiastic, because I loved his poem, and James seemed pleased at my admiration. The metaphorical representation of the "broken king" and the allusions to disaster, such as "fiery flood," and injuries seemed profound to me. This was where we worked. Everywhere you looked, you saw injury, broken lives, and disaster. Carolyn used to call our clients "worst-case scenarios." This was not, in any way, sarcastic. The things that had happened to the clients in this facility were the worst things everyone fears could happen to them or their loved ones. Working there was a heart-rending experience. If art is, in some way, the soul's attempt at redeeming the unredeemable in life, this place was the most fertile field in the universe.

Life beats down and crushes the soul and art reminds you that you have one.
(attributed to Stella Adler)

James's piece went as follows:

Broken brain
Broken king
Don't start a fire
Fire, fire, fire, fire
Fire, fire, fire, fire

Fire House
Fiery Flood
Two broken legs
Mister I did have them
Three broken arms
Unbroken neck
Sorry, New York did surrender

I was fortunate enough to be the director of this outstanding creative arts department. We had the aforementioned brilliant Peter, who was a musician and dancer, and the impassioned poetry facilitator, Carolyn, who was also a filmmaker, as well as the visionary and tireless Susan running the visual art program. The fact that we had such exceptional personnel was completely due to the company owner, who was an arts lover and was willing to pay the salaries for these accomplished, dedicated facilitators, since there was no Medicaid reimbursement for creative arts therapies.

With all this caring, driven talent running the programs, resident-generated work was being developed all over the place. Numerous residents worked on their music, art, and poetry, and some were extraordinarily talented. Others with less immediately noticeable flairs, such as James, were encouraged, featured, and nurtured, as well. In contrast to the tragic life stories of the majority of the residents, the place was alive with creative energy. Paintings lined the walls, community exhibits were common, poetry volumes were published, a CD of original resident music was recorded.

Being the serious artists that the facilitators were, this resident-generated work was highly esteemed and considered to fall within the "Outsider Art" movement. French artist and curator Jean Dubuffet (1986) coined this term (actually, Raw Art, or *L'Art Brut,* in the original French) to describe art created by those on the outside of the established art scene, such as children or people with psychiatric diagnoses. He defined it as works produced by persons unaffected by artistic culture. Mimicry plays little or no part, in contrast to the activities of intellectuals. These artists derive everything from their own depths and not from the conventions of classical or fashionable art.

People's Courage Can Be Enormous

All this work periodically came together in community shows that took place in local performance venues, and if you think it's easy to arrange community integration opportunities for high-risk, institutionalized patients, it isn't. But we persevered, obtaining the necessary multiple nursing and administrative permissions, arranging the handicap accessible transportation and required support staff, and coordinating other onerous details, pulling it off numerous times. These shows featured original resident music and poetry performance pieces with resident-designed visual art backdrops. It was a work in progress that was shaping up into a thematically connected performance piece, with the central motif being that which bound us all together: traumatic brain injury, spinal cord injury, and similar tragic fates. For someone in a wheelchair, with memory impairments, slurred, labored, halting speech, odd appearance or behavior, or obvious illness or fragility, to get up in front of people to share his or her painfully honest, soul-revealing artistic statements, requires monumental courage.

I believed James's poem would make an important contribution to our developing performance piece, so I asked him if he wanted to try to compose a melody with me for the poem. He made eye contact with me and offered his typical soft-spoken, throaty, "eh," which I took as meaning, "I would definitely be enthusiastically open to that exciting possibility."

At the appointed time, James and I sat next to each other at a piano. He couldn't tell me directly what he wanted, so I experimented with different chords and melodic possibilities. After each little idea, I would ask James, "Did you like that?" He would nod his agreement or shake his head no. He didn't concur with everything unmindfully, but clearly had opinions about what he liked and didn't like. After a while, we had our song. I played it through and asked James if he was pleased. He looked at me, nodded, and offered a slight smile, perhaps the first time I ever saw him do that.

Everyone Wants to Relate and Be Involved

We made a recording of the song. Carolyn made a film of the resident musicians and singers working on James's song. There is a piece at the beginning of the film where one of the higher-functioning residents, Alan, interviews James. He asks James if he feels good about having his song recorded, and a few other questions along those lines. James answers, "Yeah," in his shy, raspy voice—but no longer was his response simply a barely audible, "eh," but instead a more fully enunciated word. I have a transcript of that exchange and it went like this:

Alan: Do you feel really happy that we're going to sing your song, and record your song, and Carolyn is going to film it on her camera?

James: Yeah.

Alan: Yeah, he said yeah. We're gonna sing it good, Jimmy will you come sing it with me man?

James: Yeah.

Alan: He said that's cool, yeah, that's my man right there.

We made the recording, and although James did not actually sing himself, he stood proudly right in the middle of the group of singers as his song rang out all around him. Who knows how long it had been, if ever, that people wholeheartedly respected and included James as a peer.

Anyone Can Grow and Change for the Better

James's song took its place as the opening theme in our performance piece. Although he was too impaired and fragile to ever get the nursing and administrative staff to agree to take him outside of the facility for a community show, he stood with the group for several in-house shows. He participated in music groups regularly and was accepted by all present as a fully functioning member, often playing some light percussion or sitting with others as they sang. He continued to help us pack up, and rather than being a ghostly presence silently moving through the hallways, people said hello to him, with him usually acknowledging the greeting, sometimes offering a soft response.

Everyone Has Gifts

James emerged as a real-life Boo Radley (from *To Kill a Mockingbird*), whose shy, solitary ways no longer made him invisible, as his humble, artistic soul was revealed. It all happened through music. Yes, maybe there were caring, dedicated people, such as Peter, Carolyn, and myself, doing our jobs that mediated the process, but it was music (and poetry) that provided the path. Neither Peter nor I nor anyone else could have activated the metamorphosis that occurred in James simply by being nice to him. Maybe it takes a person to flip the switch, but it is electricity that lights the room. It was James's own inner light that transformed him and made him and everyone around him aware that he, even he, seemingly the most disconnected and impaired among us, was a unique individual with something important to offer. Yes, he would live out his life in this limited, long-term care existence, but his gentle, raw genius allowed everyone in his therapeutic community, the only family he had, to know him and love him.

> *This uniqueness and singleness which distinguishes each individual and gives a meaning to his existence has a bearing on creative work as much as it does on human love. When the impossibility of replacing a person is realized, it allows the responsibility which a man has for his existence and its continuance to appear in all its magnitude. A man who becomes conscious of the responsibility he bears toward a human being who affectionately waits for him, or to an unfinished work, will never be able to throw away his life.*
>
> —*Viktor Frankl (1984)*

6

Jamming

Brain scans demonstrate that brain activity is fundamentally different while musicians are improvising. The internal network associated with self-expression shows increased activity, while the outer network linked to self-censoring quiets down. "It's almost as if the brain turned off its own ability to criticize itself."

—*Dr. Charles Limb (2017), surgeon and neuroscientist, University of California*

IMPROVISATION: PLAYING WITHOUT MEMORY

Dr. Limb identifies a most advantageous neurological state for optimal music therapy outcomes. With clients in an expressing mood and reduced inhibition, they might find themselves performing beyond expectation—their own, and everyone else's. Clients grow by discovering aspects of themselves that previously were not there, or at least, not manifest. Music therapist Gary Ansdell (2005) refers to this phenomenon as people learning to perform beyond themselves, breaking out of the habit of simply being themselves to discover not who they were, but who they were not (Neumann, in Holzman, 1999, p. 129).

Jamming—improvisation—spontaneous music—lies at the heart of the Music Therapy Studio philosophy. The client is an equal partner in a collaborative endeavor of expansion of identity through loosening the bonds of ego, making manifest what was previously latent. It may ultimately be the music therapist's responsibility to facilitate the session but there are endless ways to accept, to include, to respond, to interpret. Every sound, every movement, every idea, is a potential first step into music. It starts with what Dr. Alan Turry (2016) has called "listening with reverent attention."

Jam sessions are a long-established musical tradition wherein musicians play without extensive preparation or predefined arrangements. Jam sessions are used by musicians as a social gathering, to explore new musical terrain, to develop new material, to find suitable arrangements or, simply, to play, have fun, and stretch out their chops (technical skills) without constraint. Jam sessions may be based upon existing songs or forms or may be loosely based on an agreed chord progression such as the twelve-bar blues. Jamming may also be atonal, with the focus shifting from chord structures and harmony to other dimensions of music: mood, texture, rhythm, timbre, or completely spontaneous interaction, without established musical convention, that can shift suddenly or evolve organically as the music progresses.

Improvisation has been a central element of jazz since its inception, but until the fifties, improvisation typically used established song forms and was based on prescribed traditions. In the late fifties and sixties, the free improvisation movement coalesced around such influential jazz artists as Cecil Taylor, Sun Ra, Ornette Coleman, and later-period John Coltrane. In sixties and early seventies rock music, Cream, Jimi Hendrix, the Grateful Dead, and the Allman Brothers took long, improvisational journeys. Free improvisation, as the name implies, freed performers from conventional structures, although it usually preserved one or more central elements of traditional musical form while abandoning others. In his book *Improvisation*, guitarist Derek Bailey (1992) calls free improvisation playing without memory. Bailey asserts that diversity is its most consistent characteristic. It has no stylistic or idiomatic commitment. The characteristics of freely improvised music are established only by the moment-to-moment inclinations of the person or persons playing it.

> *For me, if I don't play something that doesn't challenge my concept of what I liked before that second, something's wrong.*
>
> —*Keith Jarrett, jazz piano virtuoso (2009)*

One of the most powerful experiences I had as a music therapy student at NYU was a free jam group with some like-minded students and a professor. This group was nicknamed "The Vortex" by one of the members, I guess because once in it, we relinquished conscious control to the swirling musical and creative forces that pulled us this way and that. Once a week we went into the music room where all the instruments were and engaged in totally free musical communication and expression.

We did this on our own initiative. It was not a class. It was more like a musical laboratory where we experimented with freeing any perceived limits in ourselves within musical communication. We never discussed what we were going to do. We sang. We played. We moved. We sometimes played with a degree of expertise on familiar instruments, but just as often, we played an instrument we didn't know how to play. Sometimes, we didn't play an instrument at all. We played the floor, a radiator, a chair, or a cup. No rules. No preconceptions. No judgment. No aesthetic considerations. These were some of the most powerful musical experiences I ever had—total musical freedom, total spontaneity, total creative expression, total musical communication—or as close to that as we could get. It always turned into something wonderful, never fell flat or ended up disappointing. It has remained a seminal and fundamental experience that informs my work constantly to this day.

DAVID: THE HEALING POWER OF COLTRANE'S "GIANT STEPS"

> *I'd like to point out to people the divine in a musical language that transcends words. I want to speak to their souls.*
>
> *—John Coltrane (Thomas, 1975)*

"Giant Steps," composed and performed by John Coltrane, is surely one of the most iconic and, in some ways, most intimidating songs in jazz. Playing a competent, improvised solo over the "Giant Steps" changes has become a rite of passage for any aspiring virtuoso jazz musician. With this music, Coltrane revolutionized jazz instrumentally, harmonically, and rhythmically and furthered the development of the free jazz movement while increasing its accessibility to a mainstream audience. Twenty-six chords, ten key changes, within a sixteen bar structure, taken at a dangerously fast tempo, "Giant Steps" cycles around from one key to another with little in the way of resting points. It was so difficult that even the accomplished jazz pianist on the session, Tommy Flanagan, to his everlasting chagrin, struggled to keep up. According to legend, Coltrane had shown Flanagan the piece at a rehearsal, but he played it as a ballad and Flanagan said he could handle it. Caught off guard when Coltrane counted off such a fast tempo at the recording session, we now have Flanagan's halting, tentative piano solo for all posterity. Coltrane, on the other hand, was ready for his composition, employing a soloing style so dense that jazz critic Ira Gitler (1958) called it "sheets of sound," saying: "His continuous flow of ideas without stopping really hit me. It was almost superhuman. The amount of energy he was using could have powered a spaceship."

This level of jazz virtuosity didn't seem very likely material for me, a rock/folk/blues guitarist, let alone for music therapy, and I probably would have gone a lifetime without ever trying to play "Giant Steps." Enter and sign in to the Music Therapy Studio please, David, a 54-year-old man with a history of emotional abuse as a child and schizophrenia as an adult. A talented pianist, he attended a university music program but he was a loner, unable to connect socially with his peers. He was able to obtain his degree, but shortly after college he was incapacitated by serious mental illness that included suicidal ideation. After years of psychotherapy, he said he was not currently on medication although still dealt with some hallucinatory activity. He continued to attend weekly psychotherapy sessions and kept incredibly busy, employed as a part-time school janitor, restaurant dishwasher, and worker in a large home improvement store. He was a hard-working, serious man, extremely intelligent, with an intense gaze, who rarely smiled. Still, he was friendly, open, even a little vulnerable.

He had an electric keyboard at home and practiced diligently in his spare time (what little he had). His manner of practice was highly technical. He hadn't played with anyone since college and was not in the habit of working on compositions. Instead, he was following the curriculum in several advanced piano technique books, practicing the recommended dexterity and scale exercises. Some of them were exceedingly difficult, such as isolating the right and left hands and playing mirror image scales in a variety of patterns and different time signatures (i.e., one hand playing an ascending scale in a 3/4 time and the other playing a descending scale in a 5/4 time). David seemed to be drawn to this level of rhythmic and harmonic complexity, and this was his manner of musical relating when we first got together.

He would suggest that I join him in these exercises, but I found it very difficult to find a way to participate in this music of scales, multiple time signatures, and atonal harmonies. To me, it was all theory and physical proficiency, incredibly disciplined and impressive—but not really all that musical. Practicing scales is preparation for playing music, not the music itself.

Although David's technical capability was advanced, his artistic side had atrophied. I thought he needed to experience the expressiveness, the beauty, the collaboration, and the joy of music. To David's credit, he was open to my suggestion that we find some pieces to work on. He seemed most interested in jazz and, with Suzy, a student intern, on bass, me on guitar, and David on piano, we had our jazz trio. We settled on a couple of standards that we all knew—Earl Garner's "Misty" and Gershwin's "Summertime." We worked on them over the course of a few sessions. At first, David struggled to stay with the tunes, even extremely slowed down, but after a few sessions of practice, we improved to a reasonable, workmanlike level. It was a start, but it seemed to me we still weren't quite able to find the heart and beauty of the compositions.

Meanwhile, David continued to bring up his scale exercises and multiple time signature ideas. He wanted to try it in various ways—on the congas, then on the glockenspiel—one hand playing one time, the other playing another, tapping away without feeling, constantly shifting tonal centers, without communication or collaboration. It was all in the mind and felt isolating to me. Actually, if we were able to achieve anything like a musical unity and flow, it was because we involuntarily ended up in a unified key and conventional time signature. David didn't seem to mind this. We were jamming but it still felt to me like we were working cross-purposes and not connecting. Something was missing.

I told David that his interest in this cerebral side of music reminded me of the "Coltrane circle," a sketch by John Coltrane, famous among jazz aficionados, that reflects Coltrane's understanding of how he consciously applied the mathematics of music in his work. Music does have a mathematical component with its harmonic intervals and time signatures, and certainly David seemed drawn to this. From a clinical standpoint, I was searching for an approach that would address and shift the way David's restless quest for technical complexity seemed to isolate him. As we continued to look through books for songs to try, we noticed the chart for "Giant Steps," and since we were just talking about Coltrane, we thought we'd give it a try.

We found that when slowed down, "Giant Steps" is not so forbidding. It actually has a very comprehensible and appealing structure and melody line. But it is still quite a demanding piece of music with its rapid chord cycle and constantly shifting tonal centers. Even at a super slow tempo the tune broke down numerous times, and it took all our skill and focus, including David's, to get through it.

We stayed with it over multiple sessions and gradually we got a little more proficient and took it a moderate tempo; maybe about 1/3 the Coltrane tempo. Suddenly, David began to improvise, a bit tentatively at first, with some notes that were out of the key and out of time. But at least it wasn't a structured scale exercise. He was making intuitive, spontaneous music! The next session, when we tried it again, he did better with more feeling and fluidity. He continued to improve, and Suzy and I were able to support him in a shared, uplifting experience that stretched our abilities to the limit. I saw David smiling. It was fun!

Coltrane's genius hit the spot—the perfect blending of mathematical and harmonic complexity with beautiful music—and when we took a break from "Giant Steps" and tried "Misty" and "Summertime," again, we achieved more flowing renditions than previously. Subsequent attempts at "Giant Steps" yielded further progress as we continued to improve in managing the chord sequence and developing a more synergistic effect in our group collaboration. David's improvisations took on an increasingly adventurous, yet simultaneously, well-related quality. The grandeur of Coltrane's "Giant Steps" engaged and challenged David's musical intellect to its fullest degree while its beauty raised him beyond it, into the oneness of aesthetic, artistic creation with his fellow players.

After a couple of months, we started to get reasonably competent at "Giant Steps" with improved solos and taking it almost at full tempo. We really studied the tune, transposing it and playing it in multiple keys, creating a cycle in three different key signatures. David started to work out bass line patterns and different chord voicings. One day, I said, "I think we can take this at full speed." And we did. I was amazed! We were rocking this tune, taking solos; playing with a passion, intensity, and unity that would have been inconceivable a few months previously. We added new songs to our repertoire. David's playing had taken a "giant step" forward (if you will).

Then something even more astounding happened. David began bringing in his own compositions; some started years before and long ago abandoned. They displayed a stunning talent; challenging, complex music as striking as any well-known composer striving for aesthetically beautiful melodies and original harmonies. He introduced multiple pieces; each extraordinarily original. It was a song cycle or possibly even a musical in process. He tinkered with it constantly, each week bringing in some variation in lyrics or harmony that was different from the week before. He would play these long, intricate compositions completely from memory, recalling each little alteration he made. This was a prodigious musician at work. I struggled in an effort to help him keep it organized as it was evolving. Whether the world beyond the Music Therapy Studio will ever hear of David's work is an unknown at this time, but that in no way diminishes its grandeur and worth. I would like to help him stay in the process with his music enough to make it world-ready, so to speak, but who knows where it could land. But world or not, my job is to be a receiver, a listener, an appreciator of his music—of his truth, his soul.

Perhaps its value is simply for David's own growth. "Just think," he mused, "someone like me, with a history of schizophrenia and all the suffering I've been through, doing so well, working hard, earning a decent living, improving musically, and now, composing again." I said, "You must feel very proud of yourself," to which he humbly responded, "I guess I do. I have been feeling more relaxed because I have something inside myself that I can hold onto; that I can feel good about." When I told him it was so wonderful to see his musicality unfolding and blossoming like this, he said, "It's good to feel accepted and appreciated."

This is the essence of music therapy: creating the space and the opportunity for someone to discover and grow into dormant or previously unknown dimensions of self. That honoring of individuality while always pointing toward expansion, wholeness, and connection is the divine quality of musical language of which Coltrane spoke.

OWEN: A BEAUTIFUL CONNECTION

Believe that the rules could change. Trust that the play has great worth.

—Ron Pelias, music therapist (2004, p. 123)

Owen is my longest-standing client. I first started working with him in a parent-child group in a church basement that was my first private practice initiative in 2009. He was five years old. Diagnosed as autistic, he was not yet talking. He seemed to like music and would play a drum in short bursts of a few seconds before breaking off. He rarely gave any indication of perceiving, or being able to join with, an established tempo. Owen was able to follow along with the activities and the flow of the session with the assistance of his parent, but he often appeared disconnected or internally preoccupied, with moments of engagement and participation that usually needed to be facilitated in some way.

As Owen grew older and came without a parent to assist, he could be quite challenging. At most, his length of engagement was a few minutes, and then he would withdraw, sometimes moving away from me to another part of the room; if I followed, he would move away again. Although he made some vocal sounds, he didn't sing or use his voice in a conventional way. His drum playing was arhythmic and his instrument playing, such as on a xylophone, was erratic and atonal, seemingly disconnected to any music I was playing. He seemed impervious to my attempts at connecting. He would sometimes become inexplicably upset, weeping or throwing something, such as a drums mallet, across the room.

His parents continued to bring him for music sessions. I didn't think I was helping at all. This went on for a couple of years, with me not knowing what to do but hang in there. It's not for me to decide when or whether music will find some way to make it work. I assume music is a higher intelligence than me. The music doesn't come through me. I find a way into it. Can you see the difference? I said to Owen's parents, "I'm okay if you are okay. This is what I do." Owen's mother told me later, "I loved hearing that. Finally, someone who accepted my child in a 'typical,' yet atypical, setting."

Why should we be in such desperate haste to succeed and in such desperate enterprises? If a man does not keep pace with his companions, perhaps it is because he hears a different drummer. Let him step to the music which he hears, however measured or far away. It is not important that he should mature as soon as an apple tree or an oak. Shall he turn his spring into summer? If the condition of things which we were made for is not yet, what were any reality which we can substitute? (Henry David Thoreau, 2016, p. 177)

Owen taught me that there can be no timetable, no schedule or preconception for how it's supposed to work. Suddenly, something shifted—in him, in me, between us—I don't know. He seemed to decide that music was a safe place to be. He stopped withdrawing. He stopped becoming upset. He came to play. His love of being in music, expressing himself and connecting with me, became obvious. He didn't sing in words, although he made expressive vocal sounds. Sometimes they were pitch related. Sometimes we found a unified beat, but it couldn't be expected. Clive Robbins's term "the creative now" has never been more applicable than when I'm playing with Owen. We just jam. Moment to moment. Very free, we move in and out of tempo, switching styles and dynamics extemporaneously. It can go on for a while.

Other times, I will play conventional or recognizable songs or chord patterns with Owen, and he will do whatever he does in relationship to it. I do think recognizability and repetition is important. If the moment leads me to a certain song, melodic theme, or lyric idea, I will often stay with it for a while, just to establish a particular recurring theme in the room. He can't make suggestions, so I use my intuition. After we've done something multiple times, it becomes ours anyway. I play various songs I think he might know or like. He seems to appreciate non-Western music such as Middle Eastern or Indian (what little I know about it, but this idea is relevant to what will be discussed in the next session on idioms). If I notice Owen responding positively in some way, I may adapt the piece to include him more fully. As Nordoff and Robbins (2005) taught: the music therapist takes hold of the child's disordered world and works with this musically. Therapy then can lead the child into experiences of mobility and organization latent in the world of music. I, also, must be flexible and "in the moment" enough to experience the mobility and organization in the music. Music therapy great Dr. Kenneth Bruscia (1995) reflects on this concept:

If we are to grasp the uniqueness of each client, and if we are to understand him as a subject who has the freedom to shape his own life, then we must go beyond the laws of objects and we must begin to approach the unfathomable depths of his psyche. To do so, we, as therapists, must be prepared to move our consciousness—with courage, humility, and respect—into uncharted regions of the client's world, our own world as a person, and our world together as client and therapist. (p. 197)

Owen is 16 at the time of this writing. Although eccentric, walking backward at times and with certain hand movements only he understands, his ability to operate in the world is greatly improved. He is not verbal, but his receptive language seems quite functional. He will shake his head yes or no to indicate his answer to a question, and he will accept my suggestions of playing certain instruments together or doing things in a certain way. Usually, I play my guitar, the instrument on which I'm most competent and flexible, although I sometimes play piano and we often play percussion together. Owen really likes rhythm. Sometimes we establish a strong groove. Sometimes the rhythms are shifting, more like soundscapes than groove. We play all kinds of ways: moving around the room, hitting each other's mallets as well as drums. I express, he expresses. I intuit a groove or idiom and sometimes make up lyrics that seem to relate to the moment or the nature of our musical relationship. I stay in the *Now*, communicate, and look for signs of his communication. It can be highly satisfying, once I accept the idea that I am IN IT and don't need to control everything.

Recently, he started accepting my suggestion that he play the full drum kit while I sit next to him and play guitar or bass. For years, he would not go near the drum kit. Now that he has greater trust in me, himself, and the music, he has the confidence to take on this larger challenge. Sometimes our improvisations stretch out to a half hour or more. These experiences are miles away from his days of short bursts of interaction or needing to be across the room. I see him smile, becoming animated and engaged. It can be quiet and intimate, as well. We can sit close together in chairs or play together on a grand piano.

Owen's mother said,

Music sessions are such a highlight for him. Even after a full week of school, when I ask him if he wants to go see Rick and jam, he grabs his coat and shoes and runs to the car. The joy on my son's face is worth more than you'll ever know. Recently, when we were leaving a therapy session, my son looked into Rick's eyes with such admiration. He cupped his face, and although he had no verbal words, he expressed so much by that gesture. I cried silently in the car after we left. Someone who my son had a beautiful connection with.

Owen taught me that what is important about music is not keys, rhythms, chord structure, or song lyrics, but rather the heightened reality of nonverbal musical communication and the feeling of aliveness and connection it generates. The great jazz musician Charlie Parker said,

"Music is your own experience, your own thoughts, your wisdom. If you don't live it, it won't come out of your horn. They teach you there's a boundary line to music. But, man, there's no boundary line to art" (Reisner, 1977, p. 27).

IDIOM AND ARCHETYPE

A musical idiom identifies a piece of music as belonging to a shared tradition or set of conventions. Is it blues, swing, rock, country, gospel, classical, or Celtic? I believe that establishing an idiom as one improvises or interprets a song is an essential aspect of music therapy. Any song or improvisation can be played in any style. When an improvisation is forming in a session, I will often gravitate toward an idiom to activate increased energy and direction. I might just pick one out of pure intuition or I wonder what this music, this series of notes, this rhythm, reminds me of, and move in that direction.

Expressing various idioms or styles means discovering the defining scale, texture, rhythm, and harmonic patterns. What makes one different from another? And what is it about that particular style or idiom that one is employing for a particular effect or intention? There are virtually endless genres, subgenres, offshoots of genres, and combined genres in modern music. It is clearly impossible to categorize all the idioms in this little section. It would take an entire book just to scratch the surface. In fact, there are books devoted to any one of these styles. Of course, I am far from an expert in all these styles of music, but I know enough to perhaps scratch the surface that distinguishes the form and evokes its essence. To name a few broad categories as examples:

- Blues
- Rock
- Hip-Hop
- Jazz
- Folk
- Country
- Gospel
- Broadway
- R&B
- Caribbean
- European Classical
- Latin
- Funk
- Celtic
- Greek
- Chinese
- Japanese
- Indian
- Russian/Slavic
- Middle-Eastern

Musical idioms can be thought of as archetypes, evolving out of human consciousness and culture. They formed out of the musical evolution in different parts of the world, and their development could be traced back as far as archaeology or history would allow. To paraphrase Paul Nordoff (1998), an "Archetype" is a first form, an organizing pattern, a model, that has been transmitted through generations and becomes a collective unconscious understanding ready to be awakened. It becomes a way to touch primal identity, calling forth a response and eliciting potentials that reach beyond a client's present identity to elicit developmental potentials. In the psychology field, Carl Jung (1969) believed that the content of the collective unconscious is essentially made up of archetypes that have a divine quality relating to the source of all things. Jungian psychologist Erich Neumann (1959) wrote:

> *We shall start from the creative function of the unconscious, which produces its forms spontaneously, in a manner analogous to nature, which—from atom and crystal through organic life to the world of stars and planets—spontaneously creates forms susceptible of impressing man as beautiful. . . . And to the unknown in nature which engenders its forms of the external world, there corresponds another unknown, the collective unconscious, which is the source of all psychic creation: religion and rite, social organization, consciousness and, finally, art. The archetypes of the collective unconscious are intrinsically formless psychic structures which become visible in art. (p. 82)*

It is the music therapist's job to support the client's state of consciousness, energy level, and need for expression and communication. Which idiom would one pick for a particular situation for a particular client or a particular reason? There is no answer to that question, but one can improve in the keenness of intuition and assessment as to whether or not something is working. Sometimes, a particular idiom can really take hold in the dynamic interaction between client and therapist, even if it is unrelated to the client's previous musical preferences.

As an example, Aigen (1998) documented a Nordoff-Robbins case, Terry, whose responsiveness to Middle Eastern music was key to his progress. Terry was a nine-year-old Caucasian American boy living a sheltered suburban life. Diagnosed with autism, Terry spoke very little, was withdrawn, was easily intimidated, engaged in ritualistic manipulation of objects, and would retreat from any situation that seemed the slightest bit anxiety provoking. There is nothing to indicate he had ever heard Middle Eastern music, yet over the course of therapy, Terry's improving drum playing, vocal participation, and participation in musical crescendos indicated an intuitive engagement with this form of music. Dr. Robbins told the story that in one session, Terry actually began spontaneously dancing around a drum with his hands above his head in a style suggestive of a belly dancer. This was a child who began his first session as far away from the piano as he could get and finished up dancing and singing songs. Why should an American boy respond as he did to a Middle Eastern idiom so powerfully? Because, Nordoff responded, you're "finding the music that reaches the chord in the child's psyche—or the string that wants to vibrate, and this idiom sets it vibrating and starts the response" (Robbins & Robbins, 1998, p. 137).

Although many idioms are identified with a particular culture or part of the world, Nordoff (1998) asserts that to think of music as "cultural" is essentially erroneous, because the archetypes around which the music is formed go back so many thousands of years—actually to the beginning of time and the creation of the world (p. 137). If we regard music as arising out of the collective unconscious, all music is our common human heritage. Back in the days before trains, cars, planes, recordings, radio, TV, and the internet, maybe a particular style of music really did belong to a specific culture and place. Perhaps some might still want to claim dominion over "their music," but there is an inevitable sharing and integrating of music that simply cannot be obstructed. We could go into examples of this but it is enough to say that music is constantly blending and metamorphosing and its evolutionary impetus is not within the control of individual opinion or intention, as expressed by psychologist Erich Neumann (1959):

> *The creative power of the unconscious seizes upon the individual with the autonomous force of an instinctual drive and takes possession of him without the least consideration for his life, his happiness or his health. The creative impulse springs from the collective; like every instinct, it serves the will of the species and not the individual. Thus, the creative man is an instrument of the transpersonal, but as an individual he comes into conflict with the numinosum that takes hold of him. (p. 98)*

FACILITATING RISKY INTERACTION: GIVING PERMISSION TO EXPRESS WHAT'S THERE

There may be viewpoints one can come across in books or on the internet that contend that certain idioms, certain artists or composers, particular harmonies, even certain instruments, are more healing than others. Occasionally, one sees an article that claims something like plants exposed to Mozart thrived while those exposed to the Ramones wilted. On the other hand, an article in the *Daily Mail* (2019) claimed that one study found that plants that listened to Black Sabbath had the best flowers but those that listened to Cliff Richard all died.

As you might guess by now, I'm of the opinion that every form of music has its place. I've worked with adolescent clients who preferred rap and "metal" forms that included harsh sounds or lyrics reflecting aggression and antisocial impulses. Feelings of violence and rage are certainly an elemental—one might say, archetypal—aspect of human experience. Denying or censoring them won't make them disappear. Of course, we cannot behave violently, but is that the same as expressing it creatively? The song "Killing Machine," by the heavy metal band Judas Priest, is about a contract killer sung from a first-person perspective. Hip-hop superstar Jay-Z, whose early themes explored gritty, street-level crime, said, nine times out of ten, rappers are telling stories (Daramola, 2018). They may have seen real-life violence, crime, and antisocial behavior; things they felt needed to be expressed. These musicians may have placed themselves in the role of the perpetrator in their songs, but they weren't. It was art.

On the other hand, music can express the best of human impulses, as well. "All you need is love," sang the Beatles. Is that a reality of life we're likely to see anytime soon? Unfortunately not. Music allows for the expression—melodically, harmonically, rhythmically, and lyrically—of both positive yearnings, such as peace, unity, and beauty, as well as problematic feelings, such as violence, conflict, and despair. Such artistic impressions do not directly act out these desires, but bring them into awareness, nonetheless. Director of the Centre for Music and Science and professor of music at University of Cambridge, Ian Cross (1999), has referred to this function of music as enabling risk-free action and facilitating risky interaction. We all live with the persistent tension implicit in the conflicting impulses and dual nature of human existence. In music therapy, I believe there is no path toward resolution other than free, uncensored expression.

CLINICAL AESTHETICS: THE SYSTEMS MODEL OF CREATIVITY

The question a music therapist must ask of him- or herself is: how open am I to my client's music? This will determine what happens next. The music therapist is the receiver of the client's expressions. Psychologist Mihaly Csikszentmihalyi (1999) has discussed the Systems Model of Creativity in which there are three components of creative expression:

- **The Individual**—the artist who is using the symbols of the given domain and might have a new idea or see a new pattern.
- **Creative Domain**—that which is known and accepted in the prevailing culture.
- **The Field**—which includes the *gatekeepers* of the domain (for example, critics, teachers, industry people, the audience, and so on).

Csikszentmihalyi suggests that we only recognize the Individual's creativity when it is accepted by the Gatekeepers of the Field for inclusion in the Creative Domain. In *Clinical Aesthetics*, the music therapist is the Gatekeeper of the Field, the one to accept or reject the ideas and expressions of the Individual, the client artist, into the Creative Domain, that which is considered within the realm of acceptable music therapy (to the therapist). The essential question the therapist must use as a criterion is this: Is the client expressing him- or herself truly? Salas (1990) identified beauty in music as that which is analogous to our inner world, allowing us "an intimation of ontological purposefulness; an intuited perception that our existence has meaning" (p. 5). If it is true, it is beautiful, no matter how angry, harsh, or tension-filled it may be.

Beauty is truth, truth beauty
That is all ye know on earth
And all ye need to know

—*John Keats, from "Ode on a Grecian Urn"*

DANIELLE: NOT SO TOUGH

Danielle was seven years old. Until the age of three, she lived with her mother, who was an intermittently homeless drug addict and dealer and prostitute. Danielle was severely neglected, in addition to being sexually and physically abused during this time. When her mother was incarcerated, Danielle was placed in a foster home. Danielle's mother occasionally wrote letters expressing her intent to regain custody upon her release from prison, a prospect that filled Danielle with great anxiety and ambivalence.

Danielle had a few foster family placements, but none had worked out for various reasons. Her current temporary foster mother referred Danielle to therapy services due to escalating behavioral problems. It was reported that Danielle consistently lied and stole, both at home and at school. She exhibited violent and antisocial behaviors, including superficially cutting her foster mother several times with a knife and attempting to strangle the family cat. The foster mother described Danielle as lacking in remorse and said that she seemed to derive pleasure from doing bad things. Danielle did not deny these actions, but tended to minimize them and deflect responsibility, blaming other people (and the cat) for provoking her.

When I met Danielle, she initially presented as a sweet little girl and was, at first, amiable and compliant. She was quite musical, being able to initiate and maintain strong rhythms on a drum and create well-realized melodic and harmonic improvisations on the piano. This superficial facade rapidly faded as she became acclimated to the expressive freedom available to her in the music therapy studio. Her music became angry and confrontational. She would pound out dissonant clusters on the piano keyboard with no discernible rhythm, then abruptly stop and stare at me defiantly. Any music I made was always "too loud," according to Danielle, no matter how quietly I attempted to play or how violently she played. If I endeavored to engage in a collaborative musical improvisation, her music would become even more impenetrable, with tumultuous sounds on the piano or drum, or else she would stop playing entirely. She would acquiesce on limit-setting regarding how savagely she could treat an instrument, but she made it clear to me that she had no sympathy or caring for my needs or sensibilities. She barely knew me, she would say. Why should it matter to her how I felt or what I wanted? At one point, she emphasized the magnitude of her contempt by saying she hated me. Although I believed these feelings were real for Danielle, I also sensed that she recognized the creative forum available to her and was utilizing it as a sounding board. From that viewpoint, her expressions could be more effectively interpreted as an intuitive understanding of the symbolic nature of art, making it once removed from the directly personal, as opposed to interpreting it from a psychodynamic standpoint as transference.

Weekly sessions proceeded in, more or less, this manner for approximately five months, at which point, Danielle took off for the summer to attend camp. When she returned, she seemed less petulant. Her musicality was more evident, and she was more open to collaboration. Then, one day, after a few weeks, Danielle reverted to her earlier persona with a vengeance. Disdainful, vociferous, and inaccessible, she was in the process of smashing two hand cymbals together as loudly as she could when a screw from one of the handles came loose and the cymbal dropped to the floor. Danielle thought she had broken the cymbal (although it could have easily been repaired). Adopting the metaphorically confrontational tone that had been transpiring between us, I quipped, "Uh, oh; that cymbal cost sixty billion dollars." Typically, Danielle was astute and defiant. I expected her to easily perceive my facetiousness and reply with indifference: "I don't care," or "That's your problem." Instead, to my surprise, she looked distraught. I realized she was not feigning, as I first thought, when she slumped down in a chair and began to weep. I was taken aback and became suddenly aware of an unsettling countertransference, feeling myself a perpetrator of further emotional abuse on this already deeply traumatized little girl.

Verbal processing ensued as I ascertained the degree of her distress over her belief that she had broken this astronomically expensive instrument and her possible responsibility for replacing it. I confirmed the realities of the situation. First of all, I was joking. Second, she had not actually damaged the instrument. Third, it probably cost about five dollars. And furthermore, even if she had broken it, she would not be expected to pay for it.

When she was a little more composed, I said, "Wow, Danielle. You're not so tough after all, are you?" She sadly shook her head. "No," she whimpered. I assured her that her vulnerability was honored and safe and suggested we play "the most sensitive music we can together," a proposal to which she would have never previously agreed, but which she now accepted. I played a pentatonic scale on an electric keyboard to avoid any harmonic dissonance, as Danielle lightly strummed a guitar I had tuned to an open organum chord with no thirds or fourths. Our delicate, quiet improvisation was unlike anything we had done before. I intermittently added improvised lyrics to the pentatonic melody.

It's okay to be sensitive.
It's okay to cry.
It's okay to be sensitive
When you're warm and dry.

Regarding that last line, I felt a little self-conscious at the time, thinking I was just trying to come up with a rhyme quickly to keep the music going and that was the best I could do. It did not occur to me until later that I was singing to a little girl who had periodically lived on the street. When we completed this music, we sat in silence for a couple of minutes.

Then Danielle wanted to play another piece. We exchanged instruments. I retuned the guitar to a standard tuning as she settled behind the electric keyboard. Then she started to play a rapid-fire succession of notes, utilizing all the keys, white and black, across the full length of the keyboard. Technically, it was impressive, and there was a resemblance to her previous unapproachable music, but there was also a difference. Rather than clusters, she played mostly single notes. Although atonal and speedy, this music was still melodic and well-defined by an 8-to-the-bar, swing rhythm.

My guitar part utilized a whole tone scale and augmented harmonies to also avoid establishing a centered tonality. This music went on for several minutes and never once achieved any harmonic stability. It was wild and dissonant but was also accessible—collaborative, with a unity of artistic purpose. It contextualized her previously tempestuous and distancing musical statements without denying them, as it transformed their meaning into a boldly honest expression of unrelenting musical tension. We continued this challenging, yet unified, music until we simultaneously hit a final note. The music seemed to take a breath, and Danielle proclaimed us "Done."

Following that session, Danielle engaged in many collaborative efforts that seemed more typical for a seven-year-old, including singing children's songs together and various tonal improvisations. In one piece, Danielle played piano using primarily white keys and I played guitar, as she led us in a beautiful, classically tinged improvisation with just enough chromatic dissonance to keep it interesting and keep me on my toes. In this, Danielle also designated approximately an octave and a half on the top end of the keyboard as her solo territory, and I was to stop playing altogether when she played any of those notes. Schieby (1991) noted that any musical structure a client presents serves as a mirror of their psychological organization and, in this piece, Danielle offered a symbolic representation of a well-related individual with boundaries that establish personal space without needing to shut me out altogether. Danielle remained an intense and troubled little girl, but she had become increasingly vulnerable and honest with her feelings in music, exhibiting increased trust as she made progress in untangling her complex and guarded emotional patterns.

7

Composing

Songs are the way that human beings explore emotion. They express who we are and how we feel, they bring us closer to others, they keep us company when we are alone. They articulate our beliefs and values. As the years pass, songs bear witness to our lives. They allow us to relive the past, to examine the present, and to voice our dreams for the future. Songs weave tales of our joys and sorrows, they reveal our innermost secrets, and they express our hopes and disappointments, our fears and triumphs. They are our musical diaries, our life stories. They are the sounds of our personal development.

—*Dr. Kenneth Bruscia (1998, p. 9)*

SONGWRITING? WHAT DO I KNOW ABOUT SONGWRITING?

So said Bob Dylan to an interviewer (Zollo, 2012). To many people, sometimes even to songwriters themselves, the process of composing remains an enigma. Yet it is an integral, inevitable aspect of music and music therapy. Probably to the majority of the general public, songs and compositions, *ARE* music. In the introduction to music therapy song-book, *Themes for Therapy*, Clive Robbins and Michele Ritholz (1999) wrote that to the extent that an individual or group identifies positively with a particular composition, these pieces have the potential to play a unique role in the course of therapy, and so in the clients' lives generally. Music therapists use many types of songs and compositions. Some are written by the therapist for a specific purpose, some are written in collaboration with clients, and some arise spontaneously. Among a few categories:

- Greeting songs and good-bye songs
- Structured songs to encourage instrument playing
- Vocal fill-in songs
- Songs to express a feeling or idea
- Movement or activity songs
- Songs to encourage improvisation

Wigram and Baker (2005) have contended that the professional literature relating to songwriting in music therapy has focused mostly on clinical outcomes, to the detriment of defining methods of practice. If we agree with their point, the question arises: Is there any way to systematize a creative process like songwriting, or is it all just an unfathomable mystery? I think one important aspect of composing that relates to an understanding of the Music Therapy Studio is expressed by Bob Dylan (2012) (who actually does know something about songwriting):

> *For me, the environment to write the song is extremely important. The environment has to bring something out in me that wants to be brought out. It's a contemplative, reflective thing. . . . Environment is very important. People need peaceful, invigorating environments. Stimulating environments.*

Dylan's point says to me that the question is not how do we write a song but, more importantly, how do we create an environment that will encourage clients to feel safe enough, inspired enough, and free enough to express themselves in song? It is equally important that the practitioner have the skill set and comfort level themselves with songwriting and composition to be able to facilitate music by clients that:

- can be deeply personal.
- gives form to and enhances emotional expression.
- safely contains disturbing or opposing emotions and ambivalence.
- validates clients' inner world.
- enhances a client's ability to communicate with others.
- stimulates emotional reconciliation and self-awareness.

What is a song?

- A melody
- Lyrics set to a meter, possibly with a rhyming pattern
- Rhythmic and harmonic backing

So simple, yet so difficult. Where do we start? What decisions do we need to make as we are composing?

- What is the melody?
- What are the chords?
- What is the style/idiom?
- What's the main theme/feeling/idea to be explored?
- What's the tempo?

It's actually not that difficult. We don't have to be Bob Dylan or Tchaikovsky. A client may be able to provide a fragment of a melody or even an entire melody. They may have a thematic idea or a lyric idea but need help with meter or rhyming. Maybe they present a completed poem and want to set it to music. Most, unless they play piano or guitar, will need help with chords. Some, like Alan (in the introduction), have close to the whole thing pretty much worked out and simply need help bringing it to fruition. In a group, multiple people may contribute ideas and the therapist must act as editor, putting the puzzle of ideas together such that everyone feels acknowledged, included (see "Love Me for Who I Am"). The therapist fills in the gaps; strikes the right balance: how to help just enough but not take over.

The Master doesn't talk, he acts.
When the work is done,
the people say, "Amazing:
we did it, all by ourselves!"

—*Tao Te Ching, Verse 17*

I suppose it is possible for a therapist to write a song for a client with some clinical rationale in mind. But even in cases I can recall where I did that, the song wound up transforming to a great or large degree once in the session. The song has to become the client's song. If the client is allowed to have as much authentic input of which he or she is capable, even if the therapist is pretty active in bringing the song to fruition, the client will still think of it as being his or her song. The therapist cannot impose some external clinical conception and think that it will have any creative power. It just becomes a musical lecture. For example, I don't think it's a good idea to walk into an addiction program and announce we are going to write a song called, "Just Say No," that will outline all the bad things about drugs and all the virtues of being "clean." I have heard of that sort of thing happening. The clients may go along with it; even say they think it's a good idea. But, in my opinion, this type of dogmatic approach does no good because it does not allow the client-artist the space to make an honest artistic statement, to feel that this is truly their song.

When the client is offered the opportunity for creative ownership, the artistic process does something that can, perhaps, be accomplished no other way. According to Erich Neumann (1959) in *Art and the Creative Unconscious*, it is the product of the creator's individual psychic transformation and wholeness, and at the same time a new objective entity that opens up something to mankind that represents a form of creative revelation—a reality that only a personality creating from its wholeness is able to create (p. 166). For many of the clients with whom we work in music therapy, to live in that wholeness for a time is beyond helpful. It is essential.

JEANMARIE: FAMILY

For a number of years, I worked in a large city hospital and saw quite a few children who were victims of terrible trauma, but none more horrifically so than JeanMarie. JeanMarie was nine years old. At age seven, she was found living in squalid conditions with her two younger brothers. Rotting food, human waste, and dirty clothes lay strewn about the apartment. The only adult in the apartment was JeanMarie's mother, who lay in bed near death from advanced AIDS. No other adult appeared to be in the picture or helping out in any way. The minimum survival needs of the young children were primarily attended to by several adolescent sisters who were living elsewhere but would drop by to order take-out food and occasionally engage in sexual activity to which the children were witness. Although unclear, it is probable the children were victims of sexual abuse themselves. It was, in fact, one of the teen sisters who eventually called emergency services and fled permanently, leading to the discovery of JeanMarie and her brothers.

The children were removed from the home and placed in foster care. The mother died shortly thereafter. JeanMarie was referred to psychiatric services for disturbed behaviors exhibited in foster care, including tearfulness, withdrawal, depressed mood, sexual acting out, enuresis, aggressive behavior, and complete inability to follow directions or respond to limits. She could not read or manage activities of daily living, like dressing herself. She was selectively mute in psychotherapy sessions and exhibited bizarre behavior such as slithering on the floor. She and her brothers were placed in two successive foster homes and, both times, removed due to inappropriate care, including further physical and emotional abuse. A third foster home seemed to work out, although JeanMarie had to be separated from her brothers, one of whom was diagnosed with psychosis.

After two years of psychotherapy, JeanMarie began to show some improvement. She was referred to music therapy and immediately appeared as someone who could utilize the modality to great advantage. She was most drawn to singing, and not only was she able to improvise highly personal song lyrics quite fluently, she could also spontaneously create cohesive compositions. In contrast to her typical highly impulsive, evasive, and pressured presentation, when singing, she was capable of great focus and fearless insight although she did not appear fully aware of the poignancy of her expressions.

One of JeanMarie's first major compositions occurred approximately two months after beginning music therapy. One day, with no particular structuring or encouragement from me, she began to spontaneously sing with a voice that was barely able to contain the depth of her emotion. Although her conception of the song was clearly a ballad, she propelled herself into it with immense force, rushing phrasing, overshooting pitches, and practically screaming in parts. Her impassioned delivery communicated how important this was to her, although at the same time she was not quite in control of her artistic impetus. I attempted to show my support by accompanying on piano and assisting with the harmonic structure of the piece, but JeanMarie raced ahead of me. She tolerated me, but her hesitancy to trust me or integrate me was apparent. She clearly had an arrangement in mind, including a well-formed melodic structure and introductory section with extended rubato phrasing.

Above the stars—Someone's out there to save me
Family, family—Come and help me
Above the stars to help me—Family, family
To help me

You're the only family I need
You are out there, my only family I ever had
Family, family
You're my little brother that I always had
You are my two little brothers that I always had
You are my mother
I always help you cook in the kitchen

Family, family—You are my father
You always go to work and pick me up
Family, family—I will always be your family
and you will always be my family
Family, family—You are all my sisters
You're all my brothers

My mom and my dad and my stepsisters
and my half-brother

Family—You are my uncle, you are my brothers,
you are my sisters
And you are my cousins

Family, family, family—Come back together
We will have some fun like we used to do
Family, family—You are my best family
Family, family

JeanMarie's song simultaneously mourns the loss of her actual family and yearns for the idealized (even mythical: i.e., "above the stars") family she never had; the mother whom she helps cook in the kitchen, the father who picks her up after work. Poetically speaking, her mother really was "above the stars," since she had passed away. Her affect and imagery seemed to reflect a view of Melanie Klein (1938), wherein music is related to the integration and healing of beloved object relationships. Through the use of such musical object relations, the self aims at reaching harmony and balance by joining together psychic structures and attempting to preserve the internal representation of the beloved object. To take that concept one step further, early twentieth-century philosopher, psychologist, and educational reformer John Dewey (1934) believed that the distinguishing feature of the artistic experience is that "no such distinction of self and object exists in it, since it is aesthetic to the degree in which organism and environment cooperate to institute an experience in which the two are so fully integrated that each disappears" (p. 250). In the "Creative Now," the fragmentation between self and other, loss and desire, reality and fantasy, do not exist. In essence, in that moment, we are whole, we are healed.

As the session was coming to an end, JeanMarie reprised the family theme. She had a difficult time with endings and would fervently resist the conclusion of a session. We were in the habit of improvising a good-bye song to ease the transition, although we had not hit on a recurring good-bye song. As JeanMarie had just been singing in a gospel style, she continued with that, but instead of singing good-bye to me or to the music, she gave her final song a heartbreaking twist as she sang the following with an up-tempo gospel fervor:

C'mon put your hands together
We are family
We got power—We got joy
We got anything you need

Family
Put your hands together for the family
We are tough—We are strong
We're everything you can think of, yeah
Good-bye family . . .

As she came to this last line, I intuitively slowed down my piano accompaniment and JeanMarie slowed with me as she soulfully sang the final lament.

Good-bye family
I will always remember you
Bye-bye heart, bye-bye love
Family
I will always remember you

When we finally did establish an ongoing good-bye song about three months later, it was even more tragic. As we moved toward the end of the session, JeanMarie began passionately singing:

We will say good-bye for the rest of our life
Good-bye, good-bye, good-bye . . .

She sang the lines over and over for seemingly 10 minutes or more as she increased in intensity, even shedding tears as she sang. Bowlby and Parker (1970) contended: "Yearning for the impossible, intemperate anger, impotent weeping, horror at the prospect of loneliness, pitiful pleading for sympathy and support—these are feelings the bereaved person needs to express and sometimes first, to discover" (p. 210). After this, JeanMarie would not have any other good-bye song. Week after week I attempted to intervene by singing how I would see her next week, but she would not integrate it. For JeanMarie, good-bye was final.

JeanMarie's tumultuous feelings were often revealed in a controlling and occasionally abusive manner toward me, giving me orders regarding what and when I could and could not play, and calling me names like "stupid" and "ugly." Even at her rudest, there was a playful, likable quality about her. I did not attempt to censure this insulting and domineering behavior, nor did I react as a punitive adult or engage in a power struggle with her. Rather, I held my own and offered a stable and secure ego presence. I asserted my right to play too, despite her recurrent attempts at censoring me in various ways.

An example of how this unfolded in music occurred when I attempted to help JeanMarie tune a guitar that she wanted to play. She made it clear that she had no use for my assistance, demanding that I go away, leave her alone and, for good measure, added that I was a "loser." Affecting exaggerated outrage, I said "Loser!? I'm not a loser!" JeanMarie insisted that, my objections notwithstanding, I was, indeed, a loser. In fact, I was not only a regular loser, I was a melismatic LOO-OOO-OOO-OOO-OOO-ZER! Rather than perpetuating a verbal debate, I launched into a strong hip-hop beat on a conga and improvised my "rapped" reply. JeanMarie immediately stopped arguing with me and started dancing as a musical debate ensued.

Rick: People say that I'm a loser but I don't care—That's OK

I know that I'm really special
so you can say what you want to say
It don't matter to me—I ain't no loser
I can sit here and sing my song
She can play guitar if she wants,
but I know that I can't go wrong

Rick: I ain't no loser
*JM: Yes, you are**

*This call and response: *I Ain't No Loser/Yes, You Are,* became the refrain, going back and forth with slight variations in the wording for several minutes and returning several times during the song.

JM: 'Cause I'm singing in your face
'Cause I'm special
I'm all that you're not 'cause I'm all that
You can't sing—You can't play the drums
You can't do anything like I can do it, too

Rick: I just like to do the things . . .

JM: (interrupting) But you can't do it

Rick: Anything I like to do—I can do it—How 'bout you?

JM: But you can't play—But you can't rate
'Cause you can't rhyme—Can't tell time
Can't come on time—Always late—Can't rate

Rick: I ain't no loser
JM: Yes you are . . .

The song continued with additional points on either side. JeanMarie's fight for superiority played out at my expense, reflecting her struggle for competence and self-esteem. With her line, "I'm special," she took her cue from my similar assertion, thus utilizing me as a role model for healthy self-esteem. Other lines, such as "I'm all that you're not," also reveal her need to find a sense of competence while deflecting feelings of shame associated with trauma at early stages of development.

An important breakthrough for JeanMarie occurred a few months later with an improvised song, "Nobody Just Like You." This tribute to individuality rolled along in a sprightly folk-rock feel. I played guitar and JeanMarie danced as we as we traded lines such as:

Nobody even talk like you
Nobody even sing like you
Nobody even dance like you
Nobody in the world exactly like you

Through this song she was able to express that she was, indeed, special, despite her history as an abused child. Her willingness to collaborate improved, as did her pitch and dynamic control. Her singing became more regulated, without the frantic, desperate quality of her earlier pieces, indicating a more intact, confident presentation. She didn't need to put me down. We both could be "special."

A subsequent piece seemed to build on the foundations of the previous pieces. As I played a slow, rhythmic minor blues on the guitar, JeanMarie improvised a song with the refrain:

I Didn't Know Rick was Like This. He's Nothing But Trouble

Although reverting back to her earlier device of utilizing me as the "bad" object, she sang this country-blues ballad with restraint and excellent pitch control. Her dark vocal tone and world-weary resignation recalled blues, gospel, and jazz-influenced singers such as Bessie Smith and Billie Holiday. This piece, grieving the true nature of my flawed character, coincided with an uncertainty surrounding her adoption status and an increase in acting-out behavior at home and at school. Perhaps she projected on me what she might have imagined her foster mother and teachers (maybe even her lost birth mother) might have been saying about her. Most significantly, however, her song did not reject me. Yes, I was a lot of trouble, but she would just have to deal with it. This perhaps indicated an enhancement of her own hope, self-acceptance, and further healing related to internalized guilt and shame. The transformation of her earlier oppositional stance into a well-related artistic collaboration also could be interpreted as demonstrating a strengthening of basic trust, according to Erikson (1963), the most critical of ego strengths. For JeanMarie to acknowledge her acceptance of me, as imperfect and as much trouble as I was, would have to imply at least some belief that the feeling was mutual.

SONGS AS PERSONAL MYTHOLOGY

The underlying function of psychotherapy is the indirect reinterpretation and remolding of the patient's symbols and myths.

—Rollo May (1994, p. 342)

Music and myth both function in the realm of the symbolic, archetypal, transcendent, and imaginary. It is the role of the music therapist to assist and support the client's journey into this realm that reaches beyond the conventional and superficial understanding of things in an attempt to process and express that which seems beyond our human grasp. In this way, as music therapist/storyteller David Gonzalez (1992) points out, one can actually become a contemporary of the mythic characters of old, a player among the creators of the world: "This attitude of supreme involvement in the doing and making of the world is reflective of the stance that improvising music therapists take in charging the clinical moment with musical inspiration and relationship." At the core of mythic events is transformation, says groundbreaking music therapist Carolyn Kenny (1982), and with transformation a type of death and rebirth are always implied:

Rituals of initiation, transformation, creation, the hero myths all relate to death-rebirth. Each re-enacted situation implies going through some difficult experience, dying to part of the self or letting go of something or someone and being transformed, reborn, or greatly changed in some way. (Kenny, p. 45)

Symbolic healing is inherent in the use of mythic concepts. We connect with these universal themes in the attempt to process the events, particularly the traumatic ones, that shape our lives. The creative process, says Erich Neumann (1959), is "generation and birth as well as transformation and rebirth" (p. 202). Psychologist David Feinstein (1979) has developed the "personal mythology" construct, a five-stage model for teaching individuals to systematically examine, evaluate, and transform their guiding mythologies:

1. Identifying Underlying Mythic Conflict
2. Understanding Both Sides of the Conflict
3. Envisioning a New Mythology
4. From Vision to Commitment
5. Living from Your New Mythology

In the following story, we will see how George intuitively stepped into this mythic model to integrate and cope with a massive traumatic transformation. One could hardly say it was I who facilitated it. My role was simply to be willing to accompany him on his journey, to accept things as they were, to offer encouragement and support when he flagged and, most importantly, not to get in the way of the creative and healing forces larger than both of us.

GEORGE: SPEECHLESS

The Underlying Mythic Conflict

George was admitted to a post-acute residential rehabilitation facility following a stroke. It was also discovered George had a heart defect that would shortly necessitate surgery. Prior to his stroke at age 46, George had been a strong, healthy, and handsome single man who was employed full-time doing computer work. He was also an accomplished piano player and singer who played some professional engagements and had aspirations for furthering his career as a musician. His musical interests leaned toward jazz and classical, and he told me that he sang "like Pavarotti."

At the time of his admission, George was wheelchair-dependent, with impairments involving speech, motor skills including the use of his hands, and other complications. Emotionally, George was struggling with adjustment issues related to his condition, including depression, significant bouts of anger, frustration, and sleep difficulty. George dabbled in some music therapy sessions; however, he was embarrassed by his slurred, labored voice and typically laughed self-mockingly after any efforts at singing. His piano playing was even less functional, and he refused to make any serious attempts. George soon had to endure further surgery to deal with his heart problem that brought him very close to death. When he finally returned to the rehab facility, he was so skeletal and debilitated, I did not recognize him.

As George slowly regained his strength, he did not want to attend music sessions anymore. I maintained our relationship and continued to encourage George to resume some form of music therapy when he was ready. As we continued to discuss the matter, George made it clear that he did not wish to take part in group sessions, saying he felt uncomfortable participating with those less musically accomplished than him. That there were, in fact, quite a number of highly talented musicians participating in the program seemed to make no difference to him.

Understanding Both Sides of the Conflict

Eventually, George said he was interested in being musical again, but he would accept only an individual session. I arranged a weekly co-treatment session with his occupational therapist. The original idea was that we would work on some adaptive techniques for George's piano playing. There is evidence pointing to music as a rhythmically coherent experience of time and space, facilitating improved sensorimotor control and goal-directed movement (Hurt, Rice, McIntosh, & Thaut, 1998; Dileo & Bradt, 2005).

We began improvising in an exploratory fashion, with George on piano while I usually played bass. George would accept one other client-musician, an extremely proficient and unassuming conga player named Jose, and so we had our combo. George's OT helped with his physical positioning and some adaptive techniques. Although there was some progress in George's fine motor control and piano playing, it did not appear significant enough to be sufficiently satisfying or motivating for him. However, his musicality was soon engaged in a more comprehensive manner as George began to compose a chord pattern to accompany his improvisations. It was primarily based on a minor blues progression; however, it contained several jazzy chord changes that George said were influenced by jazz great John Coltrane.

I suggested to George that he might want to consider composing a complete song including lyrics. George liked this idea and hit on the central theme of "Speechless" almost immediately, referring to his difficulty with communicating clearly. The first verse of "Speechless" came very quickly:

Speechless
I'm speechless
I know what I want to say
but the words get in the way
And it ain't no joke when all your words get choked
Speechless

The next verse took a few more weeks. I was in favor of the song taking a wider view of George's feelings regarding his situation, but George remained adamant that the song was only about his being "Speechless" and needed to remain focused on that. George's strength of character came through as he held fast to his artistic vision, disregarding and overriding numerous suggestions and ideas by me and his occupational therapist until he arrived at a second verse that satisfied him:

Restless
I'm so restless
All my thoughts and feelings are still there
I just can't get them in the air
And I need to reveal what I'm forced to conceal
Speechless

Envisioning a New Mythology

The next development was pure inspiration. George accepted my suggestion that perhaps the song could use a bridge, and he spent a brief time in another session, the creative writing program, arriving at:

When Moses talked to God
He said, speaking for me is hard
God said, don't worry about it
Your brother will speak for you

Musically, this lyric was applied to a standard blues bridge, beginning on the subdominant chord and resolving on the dominant. But if the music of the bridge was rather traditional, it was nonetheless effective, as the power and profundity of George's lyrics gave the piece a quantum leap into the mythopoeic. George was, of course, referring to the biblical quotations from Exodus (4:10–16):

And Moses said unto the Lord, "O my Lord,
I am not eloquent; neither heretofore, nor since
thou hast spoken unto thy servant
but I am slow of speech and slow of tongue."

And the anger of the Lord was kindled against
Moses and He said, "Is not Aaron the Levite
thy brother? I know he can speak well. . . . And he
shall be thy spokesman to the people."

In discussing his imagery, George said that Moses had been one of his major heroes even prior to his stroke. The fact that Moses was someone who, like George, was considered to have had a speech impediment and yet became known as the greatest prophet of all time signified to George that his disability did not preclude his ability to do important work. George believed he had a purpose yet to be revealed.

From Vision to Commitment

When George's song was finished, he wanted it to be recorded. This necessitated moving out of the individual session format and into a wider community context. I thought it would be a profound statement for George to challenge the content of the lyric by singing his own song, but he refused. He insisted that it would sound "horrible," and no argument about how the therapy involved in singing it himself outweighed conventional aesthetic considerations could change his mind. George's choice of vocalist for the song—his "Aaron"—was Alan, another client and fellow jazz and blues lover. Alan was emerging as an extremely talented singer, although he had never known this about himself and had never sung prior to coming to music therapy sessions.

A group of client-musicians assembled to begin working on the song, with George as musical director. As the rehearsal started to take shape and then transition into a recording session, the energy and ambiance generated by the music of this group caught the attention of the facility's public relations director. She wanted to take a picture, but George disallowed it. He wanted no pictures of himself. Although George's song explored a wide-ranging coping response to his current life crisis, some of his emotional conflicts related to his trauma were clarified. A talented singer, he refused to sing (although I was able to encourage him to provide a little backing vocal part), and a proud and handsome man, he refused to be photographed. Nevertheless, the recording of his song proceeded well, and George was extremely pleased with the results.

With the success of his musical vision behind him, George seemed happier and more comfortable with himself. We began to discuss the possibility of filming a music video to accompany his song. At first, George said no, until he had an idea for an image that appealed to him—throwing a rod down on the ground and having it turn into a snake, as Charlton Heston did when playing Moses in *The Ten Commandments*. We considered this possibility, but realized we did not have the technical capacity to pull off such special effects. However, his artistic sensibilities stirred, George remained interested in the project, developing cinematic ideas and allowing himself to be filmed, something he would not permit less than a month prior. George donned a makeshift Moses costume for the shoot and later said that he felt honored having the opportunity to play Moses. He said he felt as if he connected with the spirit of Moses, who represented to him perseverance, as well as accepting the loss of royalty to achieve a higher purpose. George said, "Moses was someone who was willing to walk through the desert until he couldn't walk anymore, and like Moses, I will fight to the very end."

Living from Your New Mythology

As George began to make plans for his upcoming discharge, it was apparent that his self-acceptance and sense of empowerment were improving. He became willing to attend open group music sessions, and he sang "Speechless" and other songs publicly in groups as well as during in-house performance situations on multiple occasions. Through his CD recording, video-making process, and live performances, George came to express pride in himself and his accomplishments, rather than simply the self-derision he had shown earlier in his treatment. Although George never had the opportunity to sing his song at an outside community venue, Alan and others performed his song numerous times in concert. His recording was also played on the radio a few times, and his video was screened at a consumer-oriented conference and placed on several professionally oriented websites. His creative work took on a life of its own with his blessing as it went forward, even if he was not always present.

In preparing to return to community life, George would certainly require supportive services, and he reflected on his future and the changes he'd been through. Formerly a self-described arrogant, independent person, he accepted people taking care of him more than he had allowed before. "The World is my brother," he proclaimed. "I'm more humble and pious than I was before. It's OK that I need help. I've made some peace with what has happened to me, and an important part of this healing came from being taken seriously as an artist. I wasn't ready to sing the lead vocal on the recording of 'Speechless,' but I do hope to get back to my singing. I want to sing in local opera, who knows, maybe even the Metropolitan! I want to be the first wheelchair impresario!"

"Well," I said, "that would be about as far away from being speechless as one could go." And George just laughed.

8

Performing and Recording

WHAT YOU SAY HERE, STAYS HERE. WHAT YOU PLAY HERE, WELL, THAT MIGHT GO SOMEWHERE

A core principle of most verbal psychotherapy is privacy. The client engages in a personal process with the therapist or, at most, a relatively small therapy group, with the understanding that it will be held in the strictest confidence. This is appropriate ethical treatment. No one wants their problems to be public knowledge. However, the creative act, the core foundation of music therapy, has a more extensive intent and potential journey. In music, we move into a wider playing field beyond language, beyond personal identity and private pain.

A composer, or songwriter labors in private to distill his or her deepest essence, ideas, and emotions into a piece of music. Why? To share it.

A composer's greatest desire is for his or her music to encapsulate and communicate some universal truth that will be meaningful to someone else. Music is an act of sharing. Its deepest impetus is to connect, to let go of one's loneliness and emotional pain, not keep it private. Its desire is to assist some unknown listener to find a way out of pain and loneliness. It is an extraordinarily magnanimous, courageous, and compassionate, perhaps even grandiose, act: "People will benefit from my work. They must hear it. Let everybody hear it: hundreds, thousands, millions." When I was an active songwriter/performer, sometimes I would write a song that seemed so personal, so revealing, I would think, "I can't let anybody hear this." Then I would get over that because I thought it was a good song and I wanted people to hear it. When I sang it on stage, I realized, the audience did not know my personal situation. They were using the song as a mirror into their own soul and experience. The more successful the song and performance was at helping them to do this, the better they liked it.

HEY GANG, LET'S PUT ON A SHOW!

It is very important to stress that I am not implying that all music therapy necessarily tends toward public expression. Music therapy is complete and perfect simply remaining between therapist and client. Public expression as therapy may be unnecessary, contraindicated, even unethical, but the potential exists and is part of what music is.

As music therapists, one role we strive to fulfill for our clients—one that may sadly be absent in the creative life of a conventional composer or performer—is to be someone truly looking out for the client's interests and well-being, someone the client can trust and depend upon for support. Alan Turry (2004) regarded the client's experience of being valued and attended to by the therapist before, during, and after a performance to be more powerful than public response in helping clients to feel an internal sense of validation. Clients can be at risk for exploitation by overly ambitious staff members trying to promote their own interests and agendas. Bad "talent shows" in schools, therapeutic programs, and institutions only reinforce the image of people with disabilities as incapable, deserving of sympathy applause maybe, but not delivering anything of real worth. It is the responsibility of the music therapist to ensure that any form of public expression maintains a client-centered rationale, communicating dignity and true accomplishment for the client-performer.

PUBLIC EXPRESSION AS THERAPY: ESSENTIAL QUESTIONS

The therapist must do everything he or she can to ensure the best possible outcome and be prepared to manage the multitude of dynamics, benefits, or pitfalls involved. Utilized discerningly and with awareness, performance situations can feed back into the therapy process, but the therapist might want to ask him- or herself a few questions first:

- Who wants to perform (or record or make a film) more, the client or the therapist?
- Who's the star of the show? If the therapist's own narcissistic impulses are not fully thought through, the therapist's projections and

unmet needs can complicate the client-therapist relationship and may be, in some cases, exploitive.

- Is the therapist looking to please a boss or looking for approval some other way? Austin and Dvorkin (1998) advised that a therapist must remain constantly aware of his or her own need for recognition and validation that has not been worked through. Maybe it's an administrator who wants to "put on a show" as a way of impressing families or funders.
- What if performance is not in the best interest of the client? Austin (2003) described a situation in which her client pleaded with her to perform and later thanked her for refusing the request. The feeling of being safely contained from her impulsivity was a more important clinical concern for this client.
- Are we serving the best interest of the client's well-being? If it's a bad idea for some reason, it's a bad idea. Don't do it. Then again, you never know. It's not always 100 percent clear. It might seem like it could be a bad idea, but it's not. It's a good idea. The therapist uses his or her best judgment taking all factors into consideration (see the story of Noel).

COMMUNITY MUSIC THERAPY

We are performed beings; that is we reveal and realize ourselves in the world—mentally, physically, and socially—as performances.

—*David Aldridge (2006)*

The field of music therapy has responded to the idea of music as a "sharing art" with the community music therapy model. The community music therapy approach, according to Ansdell (2002), recognizes this essential communal reality of music-making. The aim is to assist clients in accessing a variety of situations and to accompany them as they move between traditional therapy approaches and the larger music-making community. It involves extending the role, aim, and possible work sites for music therapists. It expands the boundaries of the traditional closed psychotherapy session, but it doesn't necessarily have to refer to the conventional understanding of a musical performance.

Example 1. I worked with a former country music bandleader who had sustained a serious brain injury. He was deemed to be too fragile and disoriented to play in an outside community setting, but his former bandmates came to the institution where he resided to play with him from time to time. Although he had significant cognitive impairment, his skills, practiced for so many years, still came naturally to a degree, and having the opportunity to interact with his musical friends provided considerable joy and meaning in his newly acquired handicapped state. Eventually, he did give a small concert for his friends and family and other residents in the facility, which generated an outpouring of elation along with tears.

Example 2. Prominent Norwegian music therapist Brynjulf Stige (2002, 2003) initiated a project that aimed at integrating persons with mental illness into communal music life. Previously segregated from local band activity, they were not able to share in the musical life that may have offered enhanced membership in the local community. In addition to providing these persons the musical resources necessary to take part in communal musical activity, Stige also had to work on the attitudes and practices that prevailed in the local music groups. By initiating short-term performance projects that involved all groups, he managed to break down some of the boundaries that had kept the mentally ill persons isolated or segregated from mainstream local life.

DIRECTOR/PRODUCER/MUSIC THERAPIST: WHOSE WORK IS THIS, ANYWAY?

If we are to call ourselves music therapists, then we are not activity leaders, music or drama teachers, hitmakers, artist managers, Broadway impresarios, talent agents, or stage mothers. Sometimes, it is the clients themselves who can get caught up in the blurry boundary between public music therapy and ambition. Occasionally, after making a recording, a client will say something like: "This could be a hit!" My general response to that is: "I don't get involved in the music business. My interest is in helping you express yourself and record your song for the purposes of personal growth."

A client may be extremely proud of a successful performance or a successful recording and possibly enjoy the praise and accolades of others, but an important ethical question can arise: Whose creation is this anyway? Occasionally, clients can be extremely talented, possibly even with training or a background in professional music, but not in most cases. Although I endeavor to include clients in the production process as much as possible, I've always needed to be fairly active in bringing a project to fruition. Recording techniques that are common in the professional world, such as multitrack layering of instruments, doubling of vocals for a stronger-sounding performance, punch-in fixes for a more perfect performance, adding effects such as echo, reverb, and so on, all make for a more polished-sounding recording. A few questions arise. Is this work truly a reflection of the client? By offering our technical expertise, are we providing unrealistic feedback to the client, something like a photo-shopped image or intentionally letting a person win at a sport or game? In some cases, the client doesn't have the patience, frustration tolerance, or desire to make something so perfect, and working too hard on a project will just irritate him. The most important consideration: How is this of benefit to the client? I'm not saying that there is a right or wrong way to answer any of these questions. I'm saying the therapist needs to maintain an awareness of multiple areas of concern.

DARRYL: I WAS ALONE

Darryl was a 52-year-old resident in a long-term, post-acute rehabilitation setting. His history included severe neglect and abuse as a child, and his current diagnoses included schizophrenia, acquired brain injury from chronic alcohol abuse since early adolescence, and frontal-lobe traumatic brain injury from a car accident. He was a talented rock guitarist and singer, but his behavior and temperament were precarious. He was very easily frustrated, with attention deficits and short-term memory problems, and was prone to rapid escalation into rage, paranoid ideation, and accusatory and threatening behavior.

I tried to involve Darryl in several upcoming ensemble performances scheduled to take place both in-house and in local community venues. He agreed, somewhat reluctantly, and rehearsed with other client-musicians only to explode every time over some seemingly minor issue and quitting, sometimes a day or two prior to the concert. I was aware of my own feelings, including guilt and regret for having encouraged him to take part in situations that may have "set him up" for failure. I knew that Darryl was volatile and impulsive and had a hard time compromising his music and playing time for the sake of the needs of others, particularly when he saw them as lesser talents. I also had feelings of anger toward him for letting us down again and again.

Such moments define the "process versus product" issue of performance within a community music therapy construct. What is the primary focus, the "show" or Darryl? True, when Darryl walked out on the group, we still went on with the show. That's real life, too. But the show biz response to such temperamental, unreliable behavior might be, "You'll never work in this town, again." I never expressed any personal feelings of anger, disappointment, frustration, or guilt to Darryl. I continued to maintain my "unconditional positive regard" (Rogers, 1961), remaining open, upbeat, and positive about the future in my dealings with him. The day after one of his outbursts, I would see him and say, "How ya doing? Coming to music today?" Whatever he wanted to do, or not do, was all right with me.

Nevertheless, I continued to believe that the benefits Darryl could receive from a successful public performance were too important to abandon. I knew from many spontaneous "in-house" performances that he was an excellent performer. When he was comfortable, he could really energize and uplift a crowd, drawing many compliments. After such an achievement, Darryl became relaxed and friendly, even magnanimous, but in those situations where his music transcended his psychopathology, it was his mood of the moment that determined if he decided to participate or not. There was no pressure one way or the other; not so with a scheduled public performance.

In addition to the hundreds of classic rock songs Darryl could play based on decades of continuous listening, he also possessed the ability to improvise complete and cohesive songs on the spot. These songs were often stunningly poetic and vulnerable. However, it was very difficult to develop this new material because his short-term memory was so impaired—he could not recall the songs virtually upon completion. He seemed incapable of focusing on lyric sheets while singing, and he certainly read no music.

Even if I managed to record his in-the-moment compositions, he couldn't seem to retain them or focus on them well enough to rehearse these songs. His mood was so precarious that to push him too hard was a recipe for frustration and having him walk out on the session. One technique I hit on was to compose a chorus and a simple musical structure for the verse. This enabled me, either by myself or with others, to be the background musician(s) and singer(s), doing the recurring chorus and holding the structure together while Darryl improvised different words every time for the verses.

Only rarely were all the microphones, recording equipment, musicians, and Darryl's mood aligned, allowing for a nice recording of one of his spontaneous pieces. On one occasion, Darryl sang and played in a reflective folk-rock-soul style reminiscent of Otis Redding's "Sitting on the Dock of the Bay," and a song emerged that was essentially an expression of his core feeling of loneliness. In his gruff, Bruce Springsteen–like voice, Darryl sang:

Seems I took the long way to go
You don't know if it overflows

There's been so many times
I felt so alone
I didn't know if I was alone

There's been so many times
I've been left out on my own
I didn't know if I was here
If I was there
But I knew I was alone

I was alone
I felt just like a rolling stone
All alone

Seems so many things
Have come and gone
Come and gone
I didn't know if I was here or there
Didn't know if I was anywhere

Darryl often referred to his imminent success as a rock musician when he was discharged to the community. Whether or not this was realistic was not my concern. If I was going to help Darryl make any progress in managing his rage, capriciousness, and isolation, conditions had to be designed such that he could achieve a constructive outcome. A string of situations that exacerbated his pathology would be of no use.

I was able to arrange a performance at a local community event where Darryl could play a solo show, with me and other staff and client musicians comprising his backing group, supporting his music, his way, without him having to negotiate with others. This idea appealed to Darryl. He rehearsed diligently, developing a strong set of classic rock covers in good spirits. Privately, I hoped that the same scenario of a last-minute storm out would not transpire.

Happily, it did not, and as show time approached, we all had to manage some stress as the transportation to the event fell through and we had to scramble to arrange an alternative. Darryl took this in stride, as he seemed to find it part and parcel with being a musician needing to get to the gig. Further, the venue for the first performance was not the most inspiring situation, but we carried on in the best "the show must go on" tradition and enjoyed ourselves. Darryl played well and received some nice ovations from the crowd.

For me, his meeting the situation and managing the frustrations involved was success enough. I offered what I considered to be an appropriate degree of peerlike positive feedback (laying it on too thick could be interpreted as condescending, and he definitely would have picked that up). Once the respect and support for Darryl as a musician and a person was established, he was able to thrive in his element. He was out in the community playing his music, and he felt good about it. We subsequently did several more of these solo shows that went well. After these achievements, Darryl was willing to participate in a group project involving a songwriting session, recording session, and video shoot. He also took part in an ensemble community show, enjoying the camaraderie, praise, and appreciation of staff and his fellow clients.

Off the stage, Darryl's functioning in his therapeutic community also improved. Incidences of verbally abusive and threatening behavior diminished. Positive traits that were apparent but previously overshadowed by his anger, such as his kindness, humor, and supportiveness of others, became more dominant. Darryl became a prominent and appreciated, rather than a dreaded and avoided, member of his therapeutic community. This transformation was poignantly underscored by Darryl's sudden and unexpected death from acute medical complications. He was warmly memorialized by a large group of staff and clients. This was not a mere formality. He was, in a way, our own "star," and his contributions to the community and personal growth inspired a genuinely moving tribute to his life and music. That a man so troubled and limited in one way could still make progress and have a meaningful impact on those who knew him imbued the service, not so much with sadness or regret, but with a sense of accomplishment, hope, and love. What greater legacy can anyone leave?

TOGETHER WE DREAM—TOGETHER WE HEAL

While working at an in-patient Brain Injury Rehab Center (the same one in which Darryl was a resident), I facilitated the recording of an album of client-generated songs on a multitrack digital recorder with the above title track and album name. This took a couple of years. The song, "I Was Alone," discussed in the previous story of Darryl, appeared on this album. Each song was approached as an individual project that came up however it came up in the course of sessions. We simply collected them until we had enough to put out a compilation. Like "I Was Alone," I would characterize the songs as serious works of art—deeply honest, vulnerable, and exhilarating—reflecting the personalities and concerns of the client-artists who composed and recorded them. Some of the clients engaged in the process with a fairly intact awareness that initiated or enhanced their identity as a creative artist. Other clients, due to the nature of their impairment, were a little foggier about the big picture of the whole thing, possibly not even retaining a clear memory of the project once the session was over. Some of the tracks were improvisations that occurred within one session and would never, could never, be reproduced the same way again. Some were actual precomposed pieces that were arranged and might have taken multiple sessions to record, such as the title song, transcribed below. This song, written by Darryl and several other clients, had a rock anthem feel, perhaps something like, "We Are the World," or "We Are the Champions." To underscore this, I collected as many staff (including upper management) and patient singers as I could to sing the chorus, about fifty in all. We recorded the chorus as an overdub and for the half-hour it took to get it "in the can," we truly did believe together we can dream and together we can heal, just like the song says:

So many possibilities
So we go out in the breeze
Then we find there's no more pain
Nothing's lost, nothing's gained

(Chorus)

I sing what I believe
I sing the way I feel
I believe together we can dream
And I believe together we can heal

Together we can find a way to live
We all have so much love to give
So now my heart is serene
With the evidence of things not yet seen

(Chorus)

Whatever a client's manner of participation, everyone had a good time attending a cover photo shoot session and "wrap" party that included staff. The administrator encouraged staff to listen. The completed album seemed so enlightening and inspiring that we considered trying to enhance or remix it in a professional recording studio. The administrator knew somebody who owned a professional recording studio and we had a meeting. Although the owner was sympathetic, to his expert ears our recordings sounded amateurish. He suggested bringing in some experienced studio musicians, re-recording the songs, and having the clients become, more or less, guest singers or instrumental soloists on more professionally produced tracks.

I'm not sure where the money was supposed to come from to pay professional session players, but we never got that far in the discussion. We said to him: "You're missing the point. We can't be bringing in the ringers and slick it up like that. Perhaps it might sound more accessible to some people if that's what we were going for, but this is the clients' songs and recordings. That's the therapy. That's the point of it. That's the beauty of it." Well, the studio owner might have been sympathetic, but he didn't agree, and that ended that. As it was, the album was distributed to family, friends, and visitors to the facility. A few of the songs were aired on local radio when I was a guest for an interview. We even set up a number of local concert performances with some of the client/performers, and a music video was produced.

So what, in the end, did the patients get out of it all as they continued to live their lives, some rather discontentedly, in this long-term care facility?

SOME BENEFITS OF A RECORDING PROJECT IN A POST-ACUTE REHAB SETTING WE CAN (HOPEFULLY) ALL AGREE UPON

- Engaging in and completing the recording, then hearing the finished piece, was an uplifting, exciting, and pleasurable experience that the client enjoyed, regardless of whether he or she retained the memory of it later.
- Having the opportunity to express one's unique personal voice and vision in a creative endeavor was fulfilling in and of itself.
- Being on the album enhanced the client's social visibility and standing in the facility and led to an improved degree of recognition, positive acknowledgment, and social engagement.
- Engaging in the project contributed to the client's self-esteem and confidence, leading to the likelihood that they might be motivated to engage in subsequent music projects.
- The project was a sophisticated adult endeavor, in comparison to some of the keeping-busy activities in a long-term adult rehab center, such as arts and crafts, trivia contests, coffee socials, and bingo.
- Staff, administration, family, and friends who heard the recordings might have a newfound respect and understanding for the inner life of the resident that could positively influence future interactions.

CENSORSHIP

Once the possibility of public expression is introduced, we also open up the potential for public critique. Unlike the therapist's ethical responsibility, it may not be unconditionally supportive or accepting. Even within a closed music therapy group, there could be dissenting opinions among group members as to the appreciation of a particular type of music or expression. The term censorship, at least in the United States, tends to have negative connotations of oppressive authorities trampling on a person's first amendment rights.

The idea of censorship for clinical reasons is broadly defined by Joplin and Dvorak (2016) as the music therapist refraining from using or redirecting clients away from certain lyrics, themes, songs, or genres of music. There could be an aspect of shaping or censorship by the music therapist related to the emotional safety and sensibilities of other group members. There could also be censorship by the therapist based on his or her own opinions or sensibilities regarding the relative value of a certain type of music. This might be most prevalent with music that might be loud and harsh or expresses antisocial, violent, or self-destructive themes, as might be found in certain punk, hip-hop, or heavy metal forms. For therapists who work in schools or institutions, there could also be pressure to censor due to public relations concerns or perceived inappropriateness of material. It may be thought by the administration that a client's form of expression is somehow not socially acceptable or reflects poorly on the facility. This has occurred in my experience on a number of occasions, as in the following incident, where it was not a clinical decision, but rather outside administrative concerns became involved in attempting to manage or restrict a client's expression.

JOHN: SET ME FREE!

John was a 53-year-old man who was a resident in a long-term care facility following a stroke. Prior to his stroke, John had lived a life of minimal accomplishment and involvement, with long periods of unemployment and isolation. He sometimes held unskilled jobs such as a ticket-taker in a movie theater, and he had a previous mental health diagnosis of Schizotypal Personality Disorder. He was extremely intelligent and loved anything artistic. His stroke had not affected his speech or cognitive abilities, and he was well read, philosophical, articulate, and a good writer. However, he was in a wheelchair with partial paralysis and continued to deal with psychological symptoms, possibly exacerbated by his stroke, such as depression, social isolation, pessimism, emotional instability, with rapidly escalating bouts of rage. Because of these outbursts of screaming anger, often triggered by the feeling that he had been wronged, invalidated, or neglected in some way, he was known by the administration and security staff as prone to "behaviors." In the institutional world, a behavior never means anything good.

John was hanging around on the periphery of a music group one day when he started to grumble about how he needed to "get out of here," meaning the facility, and the staff was doing nothing to help him find community housing. His expressions of frustration began to increase until he was screaming. He was on the verge of a full-out explosive episode when my partner and I intervened. Somehow we were able to help him begin to articulate his feelings and engage his artistic inclinations. A poem began to emerge that cast him, metaphorically, in the role of a wrongfully imprisoned convict, which was how he felt. To us, prison songs had a long, honorable tradition: "Folsum Prison Blues" by Johnny Cash, "Chain Gang" by Sam Cooke, "Midnight Special" by Lead Belly, "Jailhouse Rock" by Elvis, "16 on Death Row" by Tupac Shakur. When we finished John's piece, he was considerably calmed down and pleased with his creative work. We then framed his work musically in a hard-driving one chord Chicago blues style, something like Muddy Waters's "I'm a Man (Mannish Boy)," while John passionately delivered his lyrics that he titled "Set Me Free!"

"Set Me Free!"

Yes! Stone walls do a prison make
Take the word of a prisoner
Who cannot escape from his own cage
for heaven's sake
I never broke the law
Ain't been before a judge
Have not been convicted
They got no mug shots of me
Still they locked me up
and threw away the key
The board talked about parole
And that gave me hope
But ain't nothing happened yet
Been locked up here for five years now
Gotta get my own life back
But even if I could get out now
I ain't got no place to hit the sack
Been sentenced by my life
Against my will
Got to get out now before I die in here
But I don't know how

John left the session feeling understood and happy, and we were amazed, once again, to witness the power of creative expression to transform raw, unmanageable, and deeply distressing feelings into something that we can not only live with but also actually feel good about, as if the troubling feelings were the fuel for something meaningful and worthwhile.

This is not the end of the story, however. Since the setting was a long-term residential facility, the Activity Department was always looking to find things to spice up life for the residents, and we in the Creative Arts Therapy Department often worked collaboratively with them. We had the idea to have a "Nightclub," with tables set up, cards and other casino-type games, (soft) drinks, and, of course, entertainment by several of the resident-musicians. John, doing his new song, "Set Me Free!," was to be one of the performers.

We were rehearsing for the show while one of the high-ranking administrators, a great lover and supporter of the arts programs, looked on approvingly. However, when John began to rehearse his piece, the administrator's appreciative smile evaporated, his face fell, and he quickly disappeared. We wondered where he went. We were to find out shortly when he called us to his office. He had been to see the CEO. Apparently, there were concerns that they couldn't have a resident seeming to refer to the facility as a "prison." That hadn't occurred to us. We were just writing and performing a blues song. But the administrators thought the comparison of the facility to a prison would not be well understood by family members who happened to be visiting, or worse, the State Department of Health, were they to find out. Health facilities are always anxious about "The State" that could drop in anytime for an unannounced inspection. Family and residents, even disgruntled staff, were constantly calling with various complaints that the DOH was obligated to follow up. The administrators didn't want John to do that song. Couldn't he do another one?

John wasn't a regular attendee of the music program and he didn't really have another one. That was HIS song, we argued. It was certainly "clinically" effective, having avoided the need for security intervention and shifting John's emotional state from overwrought to satisfied and fulfilled. We talked about the respected tradition of "Prison Songs," that "prison" was just a metaphor, and so on. Furthermore, if we told John he couldn't do the song, he might revert to his feelings of repression and infuriation. All the work would be undone.

The administrator understood all that, and we bandied the issue back and forth for quite a while. To the administrator's credit, he listened to us. He was such an appreciator of the music program that we finally won our point. He was willing to take the chance. John could do his song, but only this one time he said. That was the negotiation. We agreed. If the issue came up again (and there were other similar issues), we would fight another day. John's performance went very well and was a hit with the audience of staff and residents. As far as I know, "The State" was not there, and there were no undesirable repercussions. For a moment in time, John's poetic outpouring of rage and frustration and its acceptance by his audience coalesced and he was exhilarated.

COMMUNITY REVERBERATIONS

The positive side to music being identified with the entertainment industry is that in writing songs, performing, and recording, the client is doing something that's culturally idealized. If a friend, family member, caregiver, or peer hears a client singing or playing on a CD, video, or concert stage—doing something they may think only stars do, something they might think they couldn't do—that person may also think of the performer differently. In this way, the perception of disability can be transformed. It expands the context and nature of the client's personal relationships. Beyond the personal, recordings, videos, and concerts are meant to share one's talent and message with the general public. If an artistic statement moves the listener, the fact that the performer may have a disability can become subordinate to the experience of the music. In writing about the original songs on the client-produced CD previously mentioned, an article in the local paper stated:

> *The message of life is greater than the message of damage, telling us this is another way of experiencing life. We all make this choice every day: are we going to be fully alive? —Sigrid Heath (2008)*

I have had conversations with audience members following performances featuring individuals with disabilities, and the spectators have told me of the range of emotions they experience. To summarize, it begins with fear at witnessing the extent of a person's challenge. Seeing someone in a wheelchair, with slurred or labored speech, odd appearance or behavior, or obvious illness or fragility tends to frighten people because they're not used to it. As Hunt (1966) put it: "They represent everything that the 'normal world' most fears—tragedy, loss, dark and the unknown" (p. 155). Audience members may be emotionally defending against the possibility that this could happen to them or a loved one. They are ambivalent, attending the event while another part of them really doesn't want to deal with this. After awhile, fear might turn to sympathy: "That poor person—it's so sad." Then the music, the artistic expression, begins to come through and become predominant. Sympathy transforms into rooting for the performer, evolving into identification, shared experience, immersion, tears, exhilaration, passionate applause. What more do we want from a performance? I have seen audience members actually line up to talk to a "disabled" musician following a performance—someone with whom they would have previously had no point of contact.

Contemporary rehabilitation methodologies stress the principle of inclusion, meaning the individual is incorporated into the community, regardless of disability (Condeluci & McMorrow, 2004). But this is not mere bottom-line inclusion—someone in a wheelchair at a museum or social event seeming uncomfortable and out of place. This is creating a place in the culture for a person with a disability to be front and center, have their voices and ideas heard, be the very reason people are at an event. Community performance artist and activist Petra Kuppers (2011) writes:

> *Disability culture is the difference between being alone, isolated, and individuated with a physical, cognitive, emotional or sensory difference that in our society invites discrimination and reinforces that isolation—the difference between all that and being in community. Naming oneself part of a larger group, a social movement or a subject position in modernity can help to focus energy, and to understand that solidarity can be found—precariously, [and] always on the verge of collapse. (p. 109)*

9

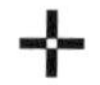

Goals

The American Music Therapy Association website defines music therapy as "the clinical and evidence-based use of music interventions to accomplish individualized goals within a therapeutic relationship by a credentialed professional who has completed an approved music therapy program." I agree with the characterization, in general, but in the Music Therapy Studio, we need to carefully consider the implication of our terms. A dictionary definition of this word—clinical—relates to the observation and treatment of disease and being dispassionately analytic. I don't think that much of what I've discussed so far can be characterized as my being "dispassionately analytic." Yes, I am making choices and doing things—"interventions"—and am hoping to be helpful to my client in some way—"goals." However, in most cases, the client is not thinking about my *interventions* or *clinical goals*. "Whether we are considering an autistic child with an affinity for playing a piano, a group of adolescents with behavioral problems creating a rap song, or an elderly woman with Alzheimer's Disease singing a song from her youth, in each case the client's primary motivation is to participate in music, not to achieve some non-musical clinical goal" (Carpente & Aigen, 2019).

Does the word clinical emphasize the disease rather than the possibilities? Do words like "intervention" and "goals" imply the passivity of the "patient"? Music therapist Randi Rolvsjord (2010) argues that the client takes actions, too, in the mutual interplay in music therapy. "In music therapy discourse, I consider the use of the term intervention to be connected to a medical model because it is a term that is exclusively used to describe the therapist's actions, usually indicating the choice and subsequent use of a technique in order to achieve a certain effect. This implies a discourse in which the therapist's actions are regarded as more important in relation to the outcome of therapy than the client's" (p. 234).

From a music-centered perspective, according to Dr. Ken Aigen (2014), "clients with disabilities and without the means to control their own access to *musicing* should have the same opportunities as non-disabled people without having to justify their access to music based on its extrinsic benefits and generalization into other areas. This generalization, although valuable when it occurs, should not be the criterion that validates the worth of music therapy for an individual" (pp. 6–7). Essentially, I agree with Dr. Aigen, but I also question how this ties in with the AMTA's assertion that music therapy entails the clinical and evidence-based use of music interventions to accomplish individualized goals. Yes, the client and I are two humans playing music. Yes, the client has an equal role in the relationship. Yes, playing music, in and of itself, can be an uplifting experience. Yet, I am a paid service provider. It's a tricky balance.

Is it possible to play music for its own intrinsic value in human life and still point the way toward helping clients discover some expansion beyond the limitations of their pathological conditions?

"The music therapist serves as a resource person and guide, providing musical experiences which direct clients toward health and well-being," says music therapist Carolyn Kenny (2002). This, as I perceive it, is my job, even if, in some cases, the client is not aware of, or even interested in, the need for such help, as in the following story.

RONNIE: HELLO, GOOD-BYE

Ronnie is a 30-year-old man diagnosed with autism. He is nonverbal. He can read and will sometimes point to a word in a book to communicate an idea or type a word or two on a computer keyboard if asked. These communications are minimal, and for all intents and purposes he does not communicate in spoken or written language. When I met him eight years ago, he was living with his parents and seemed to spend much of his day at a computer station moving endlessly from one internet music video to another. He had multiple tabs open and two screens running simultaneously. He would watch one for a few seconds, shift his attention to the other, go back to the first, change the video on one, put it into slow motion, change the other screen, and so on. His other passion was jigsaw puzzles, at which he was something of a genius, being able to complete a complicated puzzle in a fraction of the time it would take a typical adult, even an experienced puzzle aficionado. He had only a fleeting interest in social situations, perhaps briefly greeting a family friend or relative before moving back to his solitary pursuits. He seemed happy. He had a nice home, and he was loved, healthy, and well cared for.

At our first music session, Ronnie smiled at me amiably enough. He was interested for 10 seconds or so and then he turned and walked out. His mother sent him back, and he was interested for another few seconds before walking out again. If I attempted to pressure him to stay, he would look distressed, begin to groan, and take on the affect of someone who was trapped, perhaps grabbing his head in seeming anguish. And so it went. For the brief periods he was in music, he appeared to enjoy it, and as we kept at it over time, 5 to 10 seconds increased to minutes. At least we could complete one full song before he took a break. He enjoyed playing some drums and would beat away, looking blissfully happy for a few minutes before his attention turned to leaving again. I learned his preferred music, mostly American folk standards and oldies.

At first, a half-hour session with numerous exits and returns, was the most Ronnie could reasonably be asked to handle. It took a couple of years but Ronnie's tolerance began to improve, and he was able to participate in an hour-long session. He would typically walk out and be redirected back by his mother or other caregiver in the waiting area two to four times during the hour. He drummed, played melodic percussion such as xylophone or rudimentary piano in a percussive manner with one or two fingers. Sometimes, it appeared he could relate to key or rhythm; sometimes not. I created a repertoire list of preferred songs, and he chose which ones to do, often picking the same song numerous times, leaving me to decide if I was willing to go along with it or not. If I did play the same song multiple times, I would sometimes interpret it differently each time (blues, swing, ballad, rocker, etc.). Ronnie didn't seem to mind this as long as I went along with his choice.

Eventually, Ronnie came twice per week, once by himself and once he joined with another young man, Jim, who was also autistic and, although verbal, could not really have a conversation. Jim was, however, quite a good singer and knew hundreds of songs. After a while, they were joined by another young man, Daniel (discussed previously). Typically, Jim would sing, Daniel would play piano and sometimes sing. Ronnie would usually play congas or some type of percussion. This presented another challenge for Ronnie: sharing song choice. He couldn't pick all the songs and would occasionally interrupt a song that he didn't want to do by walking out or taking a lyric sheet off of Jim's music stand. Although this would sometimes break the song down, I usually insisted that we carry on. The band spirit of compromise and mutual support needed to be upheld. The "band" began to do occasional community performances at a local assisted living home. When we first started to do this, Ronnie would walk on and off "stage" frequently, but over time he improved at this as well.

Ronnie's mother reported that his progress began to generalize into other situations outside of music. His attention span could be measured in half hours or more rather than in seconds, and his ability to engage and participate in social situations, previously nonexistent, also notably improved. But despite this seemingly observable improvement, it remained a struggle to keep Ronnie interested in music for an hour. It often felt as if I was keeping Ronnie against his will, pushing him to play when he'd rather not. His mother tells me he likes coming to music, and he always comes happily. I have searched and searched for ways to engage him more fully. Often, his playing had a pressured feeling to it: banging away at the piano or drum or xylophone in a rote way, seemingly without relating to the rhythm, dynamics, or interpretation of a song. His affect would appear flat and distant, or it would become anxious and stressed looking. He often chose songs that had "good-bye" in the title soon after he arrived, seemingly indicating his desire to leave. He would look through a songbook and find a song with the word "good-bye," grab my arm, and point fervently at it. If I redirected him back into musical participation, he would usually acquiesce, but he seemed to be saying, "OK, I'm here. Let's get this over with," like I was the dentist or something.

Certain behaviors in autism might be disconcerting, such as the client frequently wanting to leave, distant or agitated affect, short attention span, holding hands over ears, or disregarding the needs of other clients. These are simply traits clients bring to a situation—not only music but other situations as well. As such, they are treatment issues, not necessarily indications that the client does not like being there. Ronnie's mother offered her view:

> *Often individuals with autism have hyper-sensitive physical senses and have difficulty filtering out all the sensory input and feel overwhelmed. The various behaviors that may appear negative or upsetting to others are a way for the individual with ASD to "re-boot," "re-group," or change focus. The trick is to try to keep this "self-preserving" behavior from completely interrupting other activities (personal communication, 2018)*

Thus, it is incumbent upon the therapist to accept the client the way he or she is and proceed from there. But just because I accept Ronnie doesn't mean I don't want to help him to play music in a more functional way. This is where the therapist's role of seeing beyond music as simply an enjoyable experience comes into play. These are our goals and interventions, and it is sometimes hard work, for the therapist and for the client. Goals for Ronnie would include:

- Increase continuity of positive experience in music.
- Increase sense of musical communication and collaboration.
- Develop instrument skills as a viable form of nonverbal communication and expression.
- Improve self-discipline and independence.
- Increase engagement in musical experiences with no attempts to withdraw.

I hoped Ronnie could discover that it feels good to connect with people and to spend a little more time doing something together. I hoped his impatience could calm down and he could find a little more focus. I hoped he would develop an increased feeling of competence and confidence in his playing, perhaps that he would conclude that these experiences are attainable for him as well as enjoyable. I hoped he could find satisfaction in being in the group with Daniel and Jim.

But Ronnie wasn't used to being concerned about his responsibility to someone else's experience. He was restless and used to doing things by himself in his own way. If we were playing a song and he suddenly stopped because he was tired, bored, disinterested, didn't like a particular song, or his attention wandered, he was not taking into account that we were playing together. He stopped because he felt like it, but there were other people playing, too—I, other clients, sometimes other music therapy students. Should everything stop because he did? Music is about communication, shared experience, collaboration, symbiosis. Every once in a while, he would catch the beat or the feeling of a song and his affect would change, becoming softer, more focused, and happier looking. He'd start looking at me and at others; the "flow" of the music would begin to carry us along. Suddenly, we're inside the music and enjoying ourselves—"the real thing," as Clive Robbins called it.

He still would frequently look through a songbook and request a good-bye song as soon as he arrived. Maybe he's telling me how he feels. People often go to work, school, even a party, with a sense of ambivalence. A musician might go to a rehearsal and wish he could have stayed home. But we go, knowing it's scheduled and we've agreed to show up. Maybe we complain a bit, maybe we'll get into it after a while. It's called self-discipline, accountability, responsibility, and we won't get far without it. Ronnie can't talk, but I think pointing to a good-bye song indicates progress compared to simply walking out on me. As a result, we've developed a repertoire of good-bye songs that are "not good-bye songs" such as the Beatles' "Hello, Good-Bye" ("I don't know why you say good-bye, I say hello"), the mid-sixties song by the Casinos, "Then You Can Tell Me Good-bye," with adapted lyrics ("We'll play our music until it's time to go . . . Then you can tell me good-bye"), and Michael

Jackson's "Never Can Say Goodbye" (with adapted lyrics). I wrote one for him called "You've Got to Say Hello before You Say Good-bye," that he liked. When he wants to leave, if I switch to a "not good-bye" song, it seems to channel, express, and discharge the energy of overwhelming feelings, transforming them into connection. He doesn't actually need to do good-bye when we can sing about it.

His drumming has continued to improve such that he can legitimately lay down a groove. At these times, he seems to really get into it and entirely forget about wanting to leave. We maintain direct eye contact, connecting on tempos, decrescendos, and ritardandos as we come to the end of a song. It is miles away from where we started. He will usually hit the last accent on a drum or cymbal indicating the end of the song.

Ronnie's mother reports that he always appears happy and energized after a session, smiling enthusiastically all the way home. Ronnie's interest and engagement in the world around him have vastly improved, such as:

- attention span now measured in half hours or more rather than in seconds (can participate in hour-long music sessions with few or no breaks)
- improvement in social interaction (such as visits with family and friends—previously nonexistent)
- acknowledging and appreciating praise now when he used to be indifferent
- willingness to try new things (previous typical reaction to virtually any new activity was disinterest and/or refusal)
- participating actively in community music therapy concerts (recently did a performance and played congas with a strong basic beat without walking off stage once)

These changes have been noted by all close friends and family members. His mother calls these developments, along with his ability to participate in hour-long music sessions and community concerts, nothing short of miraculous.

THERE IS NO SUCH THING AS RESISTANCE, ONLY IMPERFECT COMMUNICATION

The inherent tension in working with Ronnie's seeming ambivalence can be understood through the concept of resistance. The term "resistance" doesn't mean the client is being uncooperative or intentionally difficult. It means the client is being invited to step outside of his or her comfort zone and has not developed the necessary skills, confidence, or motivation. It is a given at the core of psychotherapy. Who wants to change? We want other people and circumstances to acquiesce to our will. Resistance is what we do to protect ourselves from that which we fear will overwhelm us. Freud was the first to identify the phenomenon, and strangely enough, Freud himself described his own resistance to music for that very reason (Diamond, 2012).

> *I am almost incapable of obtaining any pleasure [from music]. Some rationalistic, or perhaps analytic, turn of mind in me rebels against being moved by a thing without knowing why I am thus affected and what it is that affects me.*

Resistance in psychotherapy may be defined differently by various practitioners, but ultimately it involves a client's seeming unwillingness to respond to the therapist's interventions. Resistance does not mean the client is having a bad experience or the therapy is not going well. The therapist must continually seek for the correct way to accept, to connect, and to move through resistance without the client becoming overwhelmed and quitting. Resistance in therapy is not something the client "does." It is the product of interaction between client and practitioner. If we say, "the client resists" (or worse, he/she is a resistant client), we are giving the client the sole responsibility (and possibly blame) for some type of failed communication. I believe it is the therapist's responsibility to continually seek different, better, and new ways to communicate if our intent is not being received well by the client. Here are some other things for the therapist to consider.

Do you understand the client's interests, needs, and values?

- What are you communicating nonverbally through your music, affect, interventions, and body language? Could you be communicating irritation, control, impatience, arrogance, condescension? Perhaps you may have your own countertransference to work through, such as feeling misunderstood or unappreciated.
- What worked before might not work now. Try something new.
- Your client or the creative process may need more patience than you would expect. Authentic creative and musical communication is continuous, evolutionary, and moves toward an unfolding of awareness, mutuality, and transformation in its own time.
- Perhaps you are misinterpreting. Your responsibility as the clinician is to seek flexibility in the way you communicate with and understand your client and the ways they are communicating with you.

If the clinician practices *nonresistance*—that is, nonattachment to a specific outcome, approach, or preconception—perhaps the client will have less to resist. The key to nonresistance is for the clinician to become aware of the various forms of attachment to which one might cling and the fears involved in "letting go." David Hawkins (2006), whose theories will be discussed in more depth shortly, has identified numerous conflicting dualities (table 9.1). These would apply equally to both the clinician's as well as the client's forms of resistance.

Table 9.1.

Attachment	*Fear*
Control	Surrender
Familiarity, habit	Change, uncertainty, strangeness
Clinging to the old	The unknown or the new
The easy way	Difficult, effort
Ignore, deny, reject	Look at, face
Refuse to own	Responsibility, accountability
I can't	The truth of "I won't"
Don't want to	Can't
Rigidity, repetitious	Learn
Homeostasis, stability	Reprogram, shift, off-balance
The past as an excuse	The present as the change agent
"I'll try," "I'm going to"	Do
Tomorrow	Now
Procrastinate	Failure
Pretend	Be honest
Unwilling	Accept

WHAT ARE WE LOOKING FOR?

In my early professional years I was asking the question: How can I treat, or cure, or change this person? Now I would phrase the question in this way: How can I provide a relationship which this person may use for his own personal growth?

—Carl Rogers (1961)

Client and therapist create together. It is the music-making relationship and creative process itself that will ultimately take the client forward in his or her growth and development. Outcomes can be further analyzed to set treatment goals and evaluate progress. Typically, music therapists think of their basic Goal Domains as:

- **Communication Skills:** including improving speech and verbal communication and effective use of nonverbal communication
- **Behavioral Skills:** including increasing on-task behavior, increasing participation, and decreasing interfering behaviors
- **Motor Skills:** including maintaining or improving fine and gross motor functioning
- **Emotional Skills:** including improving impulse control and emotional management
- **Attentional Skills:** including increasing attention span and the ability to focus and follow instructions
- **Social Skills:** including improving social interaction with others, improving appropriate eye contact, and increasing the ability to share with others
- **Musical Skills:** including improving basic beat, the ability to render a coherent melody, and singing with greater volume or correct pitch

THERAPIST – 1, CLIENT – 0: DOCUMENTING MEASURABLE BEHAVIOR

These domains are open-ended and flexible enough to be interpreted according to a music therapist's particular approach. However, as music therapist Joanne Lowey (2000) wrote, other than some notable exceptions, "the majority of assessment tools currently being utilized by music therapists appear as forms with specific behavioral tasks that are seemingly unrelated to the dynamic musical relationship that naturally occurs between client and therapist" (p. 48). An example of such a behavioral goal that appears measurable and quantifiable might be: "The client will demonstrate appropriate turn-taking skills by sitting in seat without disruptive behavior and waiting for own turn four out of five opportunities to do so." Such a goal might occur in a school setting where the emphasis is on self-regulation and following instructions. Let's say the therapist is singing a song about beating a drum one time while a hand drum is being passed around. The children are expected to stay focused on the task at hand, to remain in their seat, and to hit the drum one time as it is presented. They should not jump up, call out, grab for the drum, or otherwise demonstrate disruptive behavior. If an impulsive, distractible, or typically noncompliant child is able to accomplish this goal, it is observable and quantitative and therefore ostensibly evidenced-based data. The information such data would not provide is why the child waited for her turn. Was the child promised some type of reward if he or she was good? Was the child being fed a reinforcing treat as the drum was being passed or continually reminded, or even physically restrained, by an adult while waiting? Was the child completely disinterested in the drum being passed around and simply hit it in a perfunctory way, or was his or her hand manipulated like a puppet by an adult when it was presented to him or her? In such cases, a behavior has been targeted as the "principal indicator of change . . . regardless of the process used to make those changes" (Hanser, 1999, p. 105). The goal might be achieved, the observable outcome is documented, but with potentially little or no actual benefit to the client. Dr John Carpente, a leader in music-centered research and assessment, points out the following: "The clinical significance of a musical response is not determined by the behavioral aspects alone, but by the degree of affective engagement and relational intent being expressed" (Dr. John Carpente, 2018).

THE ELEMENTS OF WELL-BEING

What is great in man is that he is a bridge and not a goal.

—Friedrich Nietzsche (1999)

I was interested in a model of assessment and goal achievement that had a universal theme, one that didn't focus on pathology and could just as easily apply to the practitioner as the client. In the Music Therapy Studio we are working primarily with clients with post-acute or ongoing conditions. What would seem to matter most is an individual's subjective experience related to quality of life. Although behavioral data may appear to be evidenced-based and modern technology has even made it possible to peer into brain activity, there remains a fundamental problem in measuring the subjective experience of another person. According to David Chalmers and Christof Koch (2017), professor of philosophy at New York University:

> *Brain processes might help us with some of what I call the easy problems of consciousness—problems of behavior, how it is we respond to a stimulus, how we can walk and talk and get around—but the hard problem of consciousness is the problem of subjective experience. Why does it feel like something from the inside?*

Researchers in the field of "positive psychology" who study what we need to thrive, rather than what's wrong with us, have identified the factors that lead to life satisfaction (Diener, Saptya, and Suh, 1998):

- Full engagement in activities
- Making a fuller contribution by utilizing one's personal strengths
- Finding meaning based on investing in something larger than the self

Large-data studies of "Flow," experiences (Csíkszentmihályi, 1990) known as "the psychology of optimal experience," have suggested that people experience meaning and fulfillment when mastering challenging tasks, and that the experience comes from the way tasks are approached and performed rather than the particular choice of task. So in terms of being helpful to clients beyond simply offering them access to music, the question for me was: How can we assess what might be important to clients in helping them to feel better and do better in settings outside of the studio setting?

The answer began to emerge when I compiled numerous personal interviews and written reflections by adult clients discussing their impressions following the completion of various studio-related musical projects such as songwriting, recording, video shoots, and live community performances. I was interested in what felt positive about the experiences from the client's perspective. All the participants had histories of long-term disabilities related to brain injury, stroke, spinal cord injury, complex medical conditions, psychiatric diagnoses, and neurological disorders. Analyzing their statements relating to their artistic achievements revealed self-assessment of a high degree of functionality and fulfillment in certain desirable personal qualities and experiences. I categorized the areas of greatest impact as follows:

- **Enjoyment**—deriving fun, pleasure and fulfillment from one's experiences
- **Affiliation**—finding ways to contribute, share, and relate with others; sense of belonging, reciprocity, and interdependence
- **Self-Expression**—feeling that one's unique personality traits, capabilities, opinions, and emotions are able to be communicated and felt to be received by others
- **Self-Efficacy**—feeling that one is autonomous and competent
- **Engagement**—being active, focused, and immersed in one's interests

It seemed to me these categories referred to qualities of inner experience that all people need to develop. In general, most fields of therapy have been more oriented toward assessing pathology rather than the factors that influence well-being, a point expressed by Maslow (1987):

The science of psychology has been far more successful on the negative than on the positive side. It has revealed to us much about man's shortcomings, his illness, his sins, but little about his potentialities, his virtues, his achievable aspirations, or his full psychological height. It is as if psychology has voluntarily restricted itself to only half its rightful jurisdiction—the darker, meaner half. (p. 354)

I compared the categories, which I dubbed the "Elements of Well-Being" (Soshensky, 2011), to other models and assessments aimed at identifying positive functioning and found correlation among all these, to name a few:

- Maslow's Hierarchy of Needs model (1968)
- Positive Psychology concepts (Seligman & Csikszentmihalyi, 2000)
- Ryff's Six-Factor Model of Psychological Well-being (1989)
- Popular articles and books about the "Science of Happiness" (Wallis, 2005; Klein, 2006)
- The Nordoff-Robbins scales
- The Sense of Community Index (a measurement for clinical practice)
- The Functional Emotional Assessment Scale (FEAS) (designed to measure emotional functioning in children)
- The Circle of Courage Model (Brendtro, Brokenleg, & Van Bockern, 1990) (integrating the cultural wisdom of tribal peoples and findings of modern youth development research)

In the Music Therapy Studio, assessments and goals are realized within the music-making process. In making the original statements that led to the "Elements of Well-Being," the clients' self-perceptions were achieved in music and were corroborated by their successful real-life musical experiences, completing their musical projects and feeling good about their musical endeavors. Within the freedom of artistic expression, one may come to understand, perhaps momentarily, perhaps more enduringly, that one thing remains forever within one's grasp—what Victor Frankl (1984) called the last of the human freedoms—the ability to choose one's attitude in any given set of circumstances.

FLOW AND THE ELEMENTS OF WELL-BEING

One model that lines up quite compatibly with the "Elements of Well-Being" is what Mihaly Csíkszentmihályi (1999) called Flow, the psychological state in which a person performing an activity becomes fully immersed in a feeling of energized focus, full involvement, and enjoyment. Flow helps to integrate the self because in that state of deep concentration, consciousness is well ordered and can become a bridge to achievement that surpasses preconception.

We are all born with two contradictory sets of instructions, said Csíkszentmihályi:

- **A Conservative Tendency:** instincts for self-preservation, self-aggrandizement, and maintaining habits.
- **An Expansive Tendency:** instincts for exploring, enjoying novelty, and taking risks.

We need both, but whereas the first tendency requires little encouragement, the second may need more cultivation and opportunity. How do we achieve "Flow"? According to Csikszentmihalyi (1988), "The universal precondition for Flow is that a person should perceive that there is something for him or her to do, and that he or she is capable of doing it" (p. 30). It is a matter of matching the right challenge for the right skill level. If the challenge is too complex and the client's skill level too low, it can lead to states of anxiety. If the client's skill level is too developed for the level of challenge, it can lead to boredom. Both of these scenarios can engage one's Conservative Tendency, or in psychoanalytic terms, *resistance*. With the well-matched blend of skill and challenge, we begin to move into the Expansive Tendency and open up the possibility of reaching a Flow state.

Table 9.2.

Elements of Well-Being	*Qualities of Flow*
Engagement	Fully involved, focused in the present; intrinsically motivated; activity is own reward
Enjoyment	Deep joy beyond everyday experience
Affiliation	Collaboration; union with others in pursuits or ideals beyond self
Self-expression	Sense of being fully oneself and utilizing one's full capabilities
Self-efficacy	Knowing that the activity is doable and one's skills are adequate for the task

DOCUMENTING THE ELEMENTS OF WELL-BEING

Documentation is required by most settings and is part of a therapist's complete clinical responsibility. In the Music Therapy Studio, in addition to creating a format for documentation, The Elements of Well-Being clarifies my own understanding of my client and how I am attempting to be of assistance to him or her. The American Music Therapy Association refers to music therapy as being "evidence-based" (AMTA website), meaning observable. As such, I added some "as evidenced by" (AEB) indicators that can relate to my clinical observations and assessment, as follows:

- **Enjoyment**—the degree to which the client demonstrates the inner experience of fun, pleasure, and fulfillment

  AEB: positive affect, positive comments, humor, enthusiasm

- **Affiliation**—the degree to which the client demonstrates the desire and ability to contribute, share, and relate with others; sense of belonging, reciprocity, and interdependence

  AEB: listening and responding, empathy and respect for boundaries and needs of others, initiating communication, collaboration and cooperation

- **Self-Expression**—the degree to which the client's unique personality traits, capabilities, opinions, and emotions are able to be communicated and felt to be received by others

  AEB: sharing of ideas and feelings, indicating needs and preferences, risk-taking, originality, individuality

- **Self-Efficacy**—the degree to which the client demonstrates autonomy, discipline, skills, impulse control, anxiety management, confidence, and the ability to adapt

  AEB: impulse and emotional regulation, willingness to try and practice, technical capability and skill, independence and choice

- **Engagement**—the degree to which the client demonstrates focused participation, interest, and intention

  AEB: active participation, intrinsic motivation and intention, commitment and closure to task and projects, sustained concentration

Within this format, here is an example of documentation for Ronnie (as discussed earlier in this chapter):

Enjoyment

Observations/Assessment: increase noted in frequency of positive affect, smiling, enthusiasm, and appreciation for music-making. Will sometimes appear stressed or dissatisfied when music is not his choice or impulse to leave is redirected by therapist.

Goals:—Increase continuity of positive experience in music especially during "down-time" (in-between songs) or during music that is not his choice (i.e., chosen by another client or therapist).
—Expand sense of fulfillment in playing an instrumental part (such as drum, piano, or xylophone).

Affiliation

Observations/Assessment: increase in eye-contact, listening, and responding musically; exhibits increased willingness to relate with others through music. Because he is nonverbal, his sense of connection must come mostly through instrumental participation and song choice.

Goals:—Continue to internalize sense of belonging and comfort within musical and social dynamic.
—Collaborate as an integral musical contributor, recognizing and appreciating his connection with others through music.
—Continue to increase musical communication (such as awareness of slowing down and speeding up tempos, finding a common tempo, and coming to the end of the song together).

Self-Expression

Observations/Assessment: shares musical preferences readily through pointing to songs in a songbook or personal repertoire list that is constantly being expanded. Improving as a musician, particularly on drums. Several original songs have been composed by therapist, and lyric changes to known pop songs have been adapted, based on Ronnie's feelings, impulses, and musical interests.

Goals:—Continue to express song preference and build repertoire list.
—Continue developing instrument skills as a viable form of nonverbal communication.
—Participate in composing, finding "voice" in original songs based on interests and personal feelings.

Self-efficacy

Observations/Assessment: appreciable increase in technical skill as a musician, particularly as a percussionist, following cues, finding basic beat; improvement noted in self-discipline, impulse control, anxiety management, and independence in moving through session with less withdrawal and increased autonomy

Goals:—Continue growth in independent self-management (such as moving through session without too much assistance).
—Continue to increase competence as a legitimate musician.
—Continue improvement in self-discipline (such as willingness to practice and participate in songs not his choice).
—Improvement in self-management of restlessness and desire to "move on" (i.e., discontinue song before completion, walk out, get to good-bye).

Engagement

Observations/Assessment: length of attention and focus continues to expand. Has increased periods of deep immersion in music as skills improve. Will typically indicate desire to be done several times per session, but is responsive to redirection.

Goals:—Will participate in full hour session with no attempts to withdraw.
—Increase immersion in musical experience leading to sustained concentration.

ADAPTING THE ELEMENTS OF WELL-BEING

If I am reporting to a setting that requires a different format than above or if I feel the Elements of Well-Being may not be well understood in a more behaviorally oriented setting such as a school, I will modify my reporting, possibly utilizing a paragraph or bullet-point style, using the Elements of Well-Being as a guide. This is illustrated in the examples below.

Example 1: end-of-year summary to the clinical and administrative team in a public school setting following six months of music therapy with a child, Sam, with behavioral, compliance, and adjustment difficulties (related Element of Well-Being area in parentheses, not included in report).

- Increased competence in emotional regulation and flexibility of behavior noted in Sam's ability to see and accept multiple points of view; notable progress in working things out, expressing himself and behaving appropriately with less reactivity, negative mood or resistance related to ambivalence over a possible stressor. (Self-efficacy)
- Developed a strong sense of alliance with therapist and commitment to the sessions. This enhanced and facilitated his maintaining respect

toward boundaries and opinions of therapist while engaging in collaboration and cooperative interaction. (Affiliation)

- Sam possesses a powerful drive for self-expression. He is creative and artistic and exhibited confidence and fulfillment in initiating and sharing his original ideas within a creative give-and-take with therapist. (Self-expression)
- There was a spirit of fun in the free flow of creative and musical ideas. Sam displayed a typically positive affect, with humor, and enthusiasm for sessions. Whatever mood he was in or whatever was going on for him in his school day, he seemed to welcome his time in Music Therapy. (Enjoyment)
- Sustained engagement within the arc of the sessions and creative interchange throughout, sometimes Sam's ideas were disjointed or incompletely explored before another idea took things in a different direction. This is an area for continued work. (Engagement)

Example 2: Goals (with quantifiable and evidenced-based elements as required by the school district for approval of music therapy services) for a nonverbal, severely multiply disabled, homeschooled sixteen-year-old girl (related Element of Well-Being area obvious or noted in parentheses, not included in report).

Improved Ability to Relate with Music Therapist (Affiliation)

As evidenced by observed incidences of:

- instrument playing such as drums or small percussion at least 50 percent of the time during a one-hour session
- sustained direct eye contact of five seconds or more at least four times per one-hour session
- indicating preference to yes and no questions such as song choice through yes/no head shake at least once per session

Enjoyment of Musical Experience

As evidenced by observed incidences of:

- smiling facial expressions at least twice per session
- increased purposeful and focused participation as in playing musical instruments at least 50 percent of the time during a one-hour session
- decreased unorganized movements such as hands to face or unfocused arm movements for no more than three times/fifteen seconds each behavior, per session

Improved Personal Self-expression and Musical Competence (Self-expression and Self-efficacy)

As evidenced by observed incidences of:

- instrument playing such as drums or small percussion at least 75 percent of the time during a one-hour session
- indicating needs/preferences by participating in song choice by head shake or smiling facial expression at least twice per session
- musical vocalizations in appropriate musical context at least twice per session

Improved Focused Attention (Engagement)

As evidenced by observed incidences of:

- active participation and sustained concentration for full one-hour session without any loss of engagement (such as becoming lethargic, unwillingness to have any eye-contact, increased disorganized movement)

IF YOU DON'T KNOW WHERE YOU'RE GOING, YOU MIGHT NOT GET THERE

That statement, to paraphrase Yogi Berra, illustrates the underlying idea of goals: making active decisions about where we are heading or where we would like to head. We must not shy away from pushing our clients toward the expansion of their perceptions and experiences. At the same time, we must not overwhelm the situation with our own inflexibility and agenda in pursuit of goals. We apply conscious intention but leave room for all the mystery and synchronicity inherent in music. In achieving this balance, we may arrive at the experiences of:

- Feeling capable
- Pride in a job well done
- Becoming fully immersed in task at hand
- Collaborating with others
- Feeling accepted
- Creating something that feels like one's own
- Utilizing one's full potential
- Having fun

These are the true elements of well-being and the true meaning of clinical goals.

10

Ritual

We relate to each other through what we share as humans. We come together through soul. Symbol, ritual music and myth are a celebration of this unity as well as a vehicle for practical growth. . . . We work on survival and improvement. This is the healing power of the arts.

—Caroline Kenny, music therapist (1982)

THE CHILDREN'S PERFORMANCE GROUP: REDEFINING EXPECTATIONS

It was decided by the clinical team of a music therapy program for children with disabilities that I would form a group of children who had the ability and temperament to develop material and create repertoire. The children chosen were aged 12 to 16 with developmental delays secondary to various diagnosed disabilities—autism, intellectual disability, Down syndrome, cerebral palsy. The children's emotional/intellectual/behavioral concerns included problems with impulse control, self-confidence, learning disabilities, social discomfort, speech impediments, emotional volatility, and low frustration tolerance. However, they were high-spirited, fun-loving children, not given to shyness, disruptive behavior, or limited attention. They loved making music and were always ready to jump in and make it happen.

Together, the children and I would choose, arrange, rehearse, and possibly compose some of this material. It was thought that this higher degree of responsibility and challenge within the sessions would be beneficial for the children, tentatively (but not necessarily) leading to some type of public performance. They met once per week for an hour-long session. After a few months of sessions, the children were responding positively and successfully to the material development aspect of the sessions and were expressing enthusiasm for the idea of performance, so it was decided that we would actually do it. The children had no experience performing, and after some discussions among the clinical team, it was agreed the most likely venue was the program's annual fund-raiser. It was thought the audience would be receptive, attentive, and appreciative. Even so, this was a major event, a formal dinner in a grand ballroom of a hotel with several hundred people in attendance (families, local politicians, and supporters of the program)—not exactly a low-pressure situation. When word got out that we would be preparing for this, several parents came to me with concern. Comments ran along these lines—my son/daughter:

- "is never going to be able to learn the material."
- "will forget words."
- "will be embarrassed."
- "will have a meltdown in front of all those people."

My response was, "We'll start preparing, but if it looks like it won't be a good experience for someone, we'll abandon the idea." I said I'd be willing to call it off even at the point of being backstage and ready to go on. The goals for the children were not modest. Although I had not yet formerly developed the Elements of Well-Being model at the time, my thought process still ran along similar lines (Elements of Well-Being term in parentheses):

- To rehearse once per week for an hour during the regular program and several additional times during the week for more than an hour as we approached the performance (Engagement)
- To find personal meaning and fun in the process (Enjoyment)
- To resolve interpersonal roles, managing the tension between collaboration and competition (Affiliation)
- To choose and learn material, develop necessary self-confidence and discipline regarding the rehearsal schedule, and manage frustration and stress (Self-efficacy)
- To feel self adequately represented in the group process and be willing to share creative input, opinions, and needs during preparation (Self-expression)

Although there were a few bumps in the road—arguments and jealousies between children, crying frustration over the difficulty of mastering the material, a few moments of insecurity, and the like—in general, the children rose to the occasion with positive moods and exuberance, and the performance went flawlessly. Needless to say, the children received an ecstatic standing ovation. The audience applauded and cheered for five minutes. People were crying. Why? Of course, they were extremely happy and proud of the children, but it went beyond that. Nobody was sure—not the audience, certainly not the parents, not the children themselves—that they could pull it off. When they did, the sense of triumph was overwhelming. It was as if they had won the Super Bowl!

There is a huge expansion of identity. Everything shifts. Now everyone is sure they can do it because they have just done it. The children's conception of themselves expands—the conception of the people around them—family, professionals—expands. It is like an explosion—like a Big Bang. Something comes into existence that wasn't there before. The parents who had previously expressed trepidation were beside themselves with joy. They were soon asking, "When can we do this again?" And we did do it again several times, always with the same success. They almost became like professionals, but nothing equaled the breakthrough of that first time.

GOD BLESS AMERICA: IT ALMOST DIDN'T HAPPEN THAT WAY

While that is a beautiful story, it is not the story I need to tell that is relevant to music as ritual. In fact, we almost didn't make it to the stage. Remember how I had reassured the concerned parents by saying, if it looks like it will be a negative experience for anyone, I was willing to call it off, *even at the point of being backstage ready to go on*? As we arrived at the hotel for the show, the children were excited and happy. As we gathered backstage, everyone was in good spirits and ready to go. Minutes before we were about to go on, one girl, the youngest, a generally positive, even-natured 12-year-old with an intellectual disability, suddenly had an attack of nerves. She started to cry and panic. She couldn't do it, she sobbed desperately. I could hear the MC begin his introduction for the group. The anticipation in the audience was electric. This was to be the high point of the evening. The magic of music therapy that everyone was there to support and celebrate was about to come alive. In that heightened state of awareness and emotion, I searched myself. Would we need to call it off? What should I do?

As it turned out, I didn't need to do anything. In fact, I really have no idea how it began but suddenly the group was singing "God Bless America." One of the children must have started it, but I didn't know who. This was not one of our show songs nor had we ever done it as a group before. Obviously it was a song they all knew because they all began to join in, and of course, so did I. With the emotion of the song rising, we put our arms around each other and sang our hearts out. With the final crescendo, "my home sweet home," we raised our hands to the air. The look on the children's faces and the energy that had been generated was rapturous. The children entered into the ritual space of the song. It wasn't about nationalism. The children inserted their own need for courage and camaraderie into its familiar, anthemic, majestic-sounding structure. The face of the girl who had, moments before, appeared to be terror-stricken, was now beaming with confidence and joy. The group was introduced, we went out to play, and the rest is happy history.

As I have stressed, music therapy as performance is not showbiz. It wasn't the success of the show that was important. It was the power that the children discovered in themselves; their courage in seeing it through to the end. Discounting the (loving and well-meaning, it is true, but nevertheless) naysayers, they confronted *life,* with all its pitfalls and uncertainties. That is what inspired everyone present. As famously proclaimed by Pierre de Coubertin, founder of the modern Olympic Games: "The important thing . . . is not winning but taking part, just as in life, what counts is not the victory but the struggle."

MUSIC CONTAINS MAGIC

In that one desperate moment backstage, the parents' and children's worst fears could have been realized, that they couldn't do it. Instead, it was a triumph. But for a few infinite seconds as we approached that treacherous crossroads, it could have gone either way. What happened? Lucky break? The great music therapy pioneer Carolyn Kenny (1982) wrote: "Some of the processes inherent in music which can be used for healing have been ignored entirely because of a strictly clinical orientation." One of these that Dr. Kenny is not afraid to identify is this—Music is Magic. Something happened that defied clinical or objective understanding.

A leading authority on ritual, Bronisław Malinowski (Homans, 1941), argued that ritual was a nontechnical means of addressing anxiety about activities where dangerous elements were beyond technical control. Anxiety stems from an inability to act. It is not the same as fear. Through ritual, we might still be afraid, but we can move forward; do what we know we must. According to Kenny (1982), "Rituals of initiation, transformation, creation, the hero myths, all relate to death/rebirth. Each re-enacted situation implies going through some difficult experience, dying to part of the self or letting go of something or someone and being transformed, reborn, or greatly changed in some way" (p. 44).

Certainly, those definitions relate to the children. What they did was dangerous and they were afraid. But they went through it and they were transformed. For the children in our story, the momentousness of the event, the rising above massive forces of anxiety, somehow "magically" caused a ritual to arise spontaneously.

CLINICAL PARADIGM SHIFT

"Every choice you make establishes your own identity as you will see it and believe it is," it says in *A Course in Miracles* (p. 621). The children in our story intuitively called on the power of ritual to make the choice to expand their identity in the direction of growth, inspiring everyone as the truth was revealed. They awakened what Clive Robbins (2004) called "the health and healing latent in the livingness of creative musicing" (p. 12). There are forces in music which can only be considered human in the largest sense of the word. "I must despise the world which does not know that music is a higher revelation than all wisdom and philosophy," Beethoven wrote (Hicks, 2014).

> *The main interest of my work is not concerned with the treatment of neurosis, but rather with the approach to the numinous. The fact is that the approach to the numinous is the real therapy, and inasmuch as you attain to the numinous experiences you are released from the curse of pathology.*
>
> —*Carl Jung in Ulanov (2005, p. 165)*

The numinous refers to a dynamic agency or effect independent of the conscious will. It can be called God or the Divine if you wish, or not, but it is some essence that is there whether or not it is apparent: our true identity. To expand their identity, to live with greater possibility, clients need to live something new. As we consider the children involved in the preceding example, each had a long-standing identity that was deeply enmeshed with their disability—what they could or could not do; how their parents, teachers, and family treated them, underestimated them, protected them, compensated for them. By achieving something more than was thought possible, a new identity formation dynamic is placed into action: a new paradigm. Paradigm relates to expectation. When phenomena appear that are beyond expectation, they might be described as miraculous. Therefore, to "expect a miracle," as they say in Alcoholics Anonymous (1978), is to place into action the higher power as called upon through ritual. It was the power of music as ritual that raised the children up high enough to cross over the forbidden zone between what was and what could be, leading to a:

Clinical Paradigm Shift

An expansion of the client's personal identity, as well as the way the client is perceived and treated in his/her social network.

III

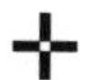

THE MUSIC THERAPY STUDIO: PHILOSOPHY

11

Transcendence

And it seems to us that one of the principle functions of all art is precisely to set in motion the archetypal reality of the transpersonal within the individual and on the highest level of artistic experience to bring the individual himself to transcendence—that is, to raise him above time and epoch and also above the limited eternity realized in any limited archetypal form—to lead him to the radiant dynamic that is at the heart of the world.

—*Erich Newmann (1959, p. 106)*

I have been arguing throughout this book about the importance of maintaining a respectful, admiring attitude toward our clients rather than that of simply being a caring provider for the less fortunate in the lottery of life. As we have seen in the previous sections, family members, friends, the general public, as well as practitioners themselves may well underestimate a disabled person's capability. A therapist's *only* job is to assist in the client's personal growth, functional improvement, and sense of well-being. Must we not, as helping professionals, be capable of remaining open to that which is not yet manifest? If not, even seemingly the kindest, most well-meaning person may keep another imprisoned by the content and quality of one's thoughts, a sentiment echoed by Goethe (1824): "When we take people merely as they are, we make them worse; when we treat them as if they were what they should be, we improve them as far as they can be improved" (p. 194).

As such, whether shared or not, a practitioner's thoughts, the way we comprehend and interpret our work, impacts the effectiveness of the session. In the most literal sense, thought creates reality. Celebrated physicists of the twentieth century such as Albert Einstein, Werner Heisenberg, John Wheeler, David Bohm, Erwin Schrodinger, and Neils Bohr have demonstrated that on the quantum (subatomic particle) level, everything in the universe is interdependent and nothing is actually separate from anything else. This theory is called nonlocality. J. S. Bell, a Swiss physicist, provided mathematical proof of nonlocality (Josephson & Pallikari, 1991) and French physicist Alain Aspect's "Bell Test Experiments" (1982) found that the communication between subatomic particles is faster than the speed of light, virtually instantaneous, in fact, across vast cosmic distances without any obvious mechanism for communication between the two locations. This effect, called quantum entanglement, has been studied extensively and found to be indisputable (Merali, 2015). Everything is an unbroken wholeness as postulated by eminent physicist David Bohm (1980). It is a level of reality that he called the "Implicate Order," wherein wholeness is not a static oneness, but a dynamic wholeness-in-motion in which *everything* moves together. As to whether one's thoughts, choices, and assessments affect this wholeness-in-motion, let us consider the famous double-slit experiment, well, famous among physics aficionados.

THE FAMOUS DOUBLE-SLIT EXPERIMENT

Does light move as a continuous wave or a shower of photons (light particles)? The answer, you may know, is both, as proposed by Einstein (Isaacson, 2007). Neither answer fully explains the phenomena of light, but together they do, creating two contradictory pictures of reality. When waves intersect, they create interference patterns, such as ripples in a pond crashing into each other. Particles would not typically interfere with each other because their path is a straight vector, such as bullets shot at a target.

In the double-slit experiment, photons are shot randomly, one by one, at a screen containing two narrow slits. A detection screen is set up behind to display the position and pattern of the photons that pass through the slits. One would expect some to hit the first screen while others pass through one slit or the other and imprint on the detection screen behind. And when the experimenters monitor which slit each photon passes through, that is exactly what they find.

Of course, in our everyday experience, we don't perceive individual light particles. Imagine, under normal circumstances, shining a flashlight at a screen with two slits. Again, some of the light will shine on the first screen and not get through. The light that passes through the two slits will split into two waves, each spreading out from the slit it passed through.

Where the two waves overlap, they will form an interference pattern on the detection screen. That seems comprehensible enough. Now we move into spooky territory.

If the paths of the individually shot photons are not monitored, that is, if it is set up so that the experimenter does not know which slit the photons pass through, an interference pattern will form as the individual photon shots build up on the detection screen. Even if the photon shots are spaced so that they can't possibly directly interfere with each other, they will form an interference pattern as if they were a continuous wave. In other words, if the path of the photons is measured, they appear as particles on the detection screen. If the paths are not measured and only analyzed later, they appear as if a wave passing through the two slits and forming an interference pattern. Even a single unmeasured photon will appear to have passed through both slits simultaneously, acting like a wave and interfering with itself. Unobserved particles seem to inhabit all possibilities. Understand the gist of this: "The same starting circumstances—a stream of individually randomly shot photons—with different outcomes—light behaving as a particle or a wave, and the only variable is the choice of active participation or non-participation of the experimenters."

AND THAT'S NOT ALL

"But wait! There's more!" as the announcer says on the late-night TV commercial. This experiment has been performed numerous times over many years with various modifications, such as the "Quantum Eraser" (Ananthaswamy, 2018), in which it was noticed that if the experimenters took the data, they saw the expected particle pattern. However, if they took the data but then deleted it before observing the results, they saw an interference pattern!

In the most astounding variation of all, celebrated American physicist John Wheeler proposed "The Delayed Choice Experiment" (Manning et al., 2015). In this experiment, the decision whether or not to monitor the photon path is made *after* they have already been emitted. When the outcome was revealed, the photons were found to have behaved as if the choice was made prior to being shot—meaning that if the experimenters chose to monitor its path, the photon behaved particle-like—no interference pattern. If they chose not to monitor, there was an interference pattern.

How can the outcome of an event already underway be affected, seemingly retroactively, by thought alone? Is the physical reality of the photon (particle or wave) being determined backward in time? Wheeler's unavoidable conclusion was this:

Reality Is Created by Observers

Wheeler coined the term "Participatory Anthropic Principle," meaning it is a participatory universe (Folger, 2002). We are interacting with it, not simply observing it. Observer and observed form an indissoluble whole that functions outside the boundaries of time. Wheeler believed that the universe is an enormous feedback loop in which we contribute to the ongoing creation of not only the present and the future but the past as well. That it can seem impossible to eliminate a decisive role for our conscious intervention in the outcome of experiments drove physicist Eugene Wigner to the conclusion that the mind itself causes the "collapse" that turns a wave into a particle. Quantum physicist Dr. Amit Goswami (2013) further explained:

> *There is no manifest quantum object until we see it, even if the object is the entire cosmos. There is no manifest cosmos—only possibilities—until the first sentient being (presumably, the first living cell) observes the universe. . . . And the observation is self-referential—the sentience of the first living cell is co-created along with the universe. . . . The point to realize is that in quantum physics there is neither space nor time until consciousness has chosen to collapse an event. (p. 43)*

A variable that did not previously exist, influencing universal evolution, is introduced the moment a conscious entity "collapses an event," that is, makes a choice out of infinite possibilities. And as John Wheeler and Bohm have suggested, everything is related—past, present and future—including the subtle energy of conscious thought. While a mechanical view of the universe, one event causing and following another within linear time and space, operating independently of observation, seems to be reality, it is not. It is only the way our brains interpret and make sense of our experience. Science, like mysticism before it, is leading us beyond that paradigm. Measurement is everything, said Associate Professor Andrew Truscott (2015) from the Australian National University Research School of Physics and Engineering. At the quantum level, reality does not exist if you are not looking at it.

> *Mind is the Forerunner of All Things.*
>
> —*Buddha*

FAR OUT, MAN, BUT WHAT DOES THIS HAVE TO DO WITH MUSIC THERAPY?

I offer these theories and mysteries, "submitted for your approval" as Rod Serling used to say in *The Twilight Zone*, to suggest that one's private inner world, one's very thoughts—what one chooses to pay attention to and collect data about, what one accepts, what one discounts, one's biases, one's assumptions, how one chooses to set things up, what one believes and doesn't believe can or will happen—all of these effect the nature of outcomes—meaning, in plain and simple language, how helpful we can be to our clients.

As the double-slit experiment indicates, the wonder of a stream of photons creating a seemingly impossible interference pattern only happens when they are not observed, not measured. Maybe when we look too closely, when we bring all kinds of notions, predictions, theories, and ambitions to a creative situation, we block that which is beyond our limited preconception. "Striving is always looking," says Goswami (2013). Therefore, he advises: "Process, don't look. Unconscious processing lets us accumulate and proliferate ambiguity through the quantum dynamics" (p. 191). Which is to say: Stay in the "Creative Now."

ATTRACTOR PATTERNS

As we know, human interactions and behaviors are complex, unpredictable, and difficult to manage. Chaos theorists who study complex dynamic systems, such as weather patterns or crowd behavior, have identified underlying patterns they call "Attractors." The theory holds that complex systems run through a cycle and achieve equilibrium for a period. The approach to equilibrium where the data coalesces and suggests the direction toward which a complex system may evolve is called an *Attractor*.

The premise of the previous section—that consciousness is inextricably involved with phenomena—sets the stage for research conducted by David Hawkins (1995) that concluded that thoughts, as subtle forms of nonphysical energy, function as "Attractors," generated by each individual's ongoing thought stream. It is as a result of these energy fields that you view the world the way you do, and these fields are why you have the attitudes and reactions toward life that you do.

Hawkins's research indicated that Attractor Patterns influence all living things the same way: loving thoughts are life promoting and negative thoughts are life impairing. Thought-generated energy fields not only affect one's own reality, mood, health, and actions, but also interact with the energy fields of others. The energy field of loving people elevates the energy level of those around them. The energy field of controlling, fearful people depresses the energy level of those around them. As suggested by theories of nonlocality previously discussed, Attractor Patterns affect not only our immediate reality but all life and existence. The energy generated by the thought streams of all entities on Earth (and possibly beyond, but we can't go there), creates the Attractor Pattern toward which the whole system of consciousness moves. As we have discussed, in quantum reality, there are no certainties, only probabilities. The Attractor Pattern acts as the underlying pattern or outlook that pulls from infinite possibility and coalesces into the world of Observable Events. As John Wheeler concluded, "No phenomenon is a phenomenon until it is an observed phenomenon."

According to Hawkins, you cannot avoid creating attractors. They are the result of the process of thinking. You can only help by increasing your awareness in order to shift your thought patterns toward higher states of consciousness.

DAVID HAWKINS'S LEVELS OF CONSCIOUSNESS (1995)

(Attractor Patterns—from the most harmful toward the most beneficial)

- **Shame**—self-blame, self-hatred; suicidal ideation.
- **Guilt**—unable to forgive oneself for past transgressions.
- **Apathy**—hopelessness; despair; no reason to act.
- **Grief**—regret; feelings of loss and despondence.
- **Fear**—seeing the world as dangerous and unsafe.
- **Desire**—addiction; craving; need for money, approval, power, fame.
- **Anger**—strong hate and frustration; often from struggles at the lower levels; can spur one toward action at higher levels, or it can keep one stuck in hatred and lower levels.
- **Pride**—one starts to feel good, but it's dependent on external circumstances such as money, power, status, and so on; a person can be so closely enmeshed in their beliefs that they see an attack on their beliefs as an attack on themselves.
- **Courage**—first level of true power; valuing truth over falsehood; integrity instead of temporary gain; able to face, cope with, and handle things better; still experiencing the lesser negative feelings but with greater ability to handle those energies.

- **Neutrality**—self-trust; brings release from painful emotions as well as letting go of resistance, which brings a lot more power.
- **Willingness**—saying yes to life; to join; to agree, to commit and align with others; the introduction of intention.
- **Acceptance**—transformation in consciousness to understanding that we are the source of our own happiness; not blaming others or circumstances for challenges.
- **Reason**—transcending narcissistic/emotional distortions characteristic of immaturity; increased reality testing and nonemotional respect for truth; the level of medicine and science.
- **Love**—permanent understanding of one's connectedness with all that exists; a deep sense of compassion; awakening to one's true purpose, uncorrupted by the desires of the ego; service to humanity and feeling guided by a force greater than oneself.
- **Joy**—ultimate state of pervasive happiness; the level of advanced spiritual teachers guided by synchronicity and intuition; no need to set goals and make detailed plans; the expansion of consciousness allows one to operate at a much higher level.
- **Peace**—supreme transcendence; reached only by one person in 10 million.
- **Enlightenment**—highest level of human consciousness; where humanity blends with divinity.

I'M PICKING UP GOOD VIBRATIONS: PRACTICAL APPLICATIONS FOR MUSIC THERAPY

Each individual composes the music of his own life. . . . If he can quicken the feeling of another to joy or to gratitude, by that much he adds to his own life; he becomes himself by that much more alive. Whether conscious of it or not, his thought is affected for the better by the joy or gratitude of another, and his power and vitality increase thereby, and the music of his life grows more in harmony.

—Hazrat Inayat Khan (1983, p. 134)

If we consider the Body-Mind-Spirit model of the whole person, we can classify Hawkins's Levels of Consciousness as belonging more to one area than another. All of these energies are operational, in one way or another, when we are engaged in music therapy. Body represents survival and separateness—me versus the other—comparison, competition, threat, control, wanting, longing, winning/losing. Mind is able to evaluate, decide how best to proceed, and make choices, despite the influence of Body identification. Mind cannot bring us into the realm of Spirit. Music, however, can.

Spirit
love, joy, peace, enlightenment

Mind
courage, neutrality, willingness,
acceptance, reason

Body
shame, guilt, apathy, grief, fear,
desire, anger, pride

In order to endeavor shifting toward higher states of consciousness, it would be beneficial to maintain awareness of our thought patterns. David Bohm, whose theory of the "Implicate Order" we have just considered, was very influenced by the work of spiritual master Krishnamurti, and they engaged in some well-known dialogues (Krishnamurti & Bohm, 1999). Regarding Krishnamurti's view of the general disorder and confusion that pervades the consciousness of most people, Bohm wrote:

> *It is here that I encountered what I feel to be Krishnamurti's major discovery. What he was seriously proposing is that all this disorder, which is the root cause of such widespread sorrow and misery, and which prevents human beings from properly working together, has its root in the fact that we are ignorant of the general nature of our own processes of thought. Or to put it differently it may be said that we do not see what is actually happening, when we are engaged in the activity of thinking. Through close attention to and observation of this activity of thought, Krishnamurti feels that he directly perceives that thought is a material process, which is going on inside of the human being in the brain and nervous system as a whole. (Krishnamurti & Bohm, 1999, p. viii)*

What would be a practical application of bringing attention to and observation of the activity of thought for a music therapy session? Hypothetically, let's say I'm preparing to begin a session and I'm dealing with a lower state of consciousness, perhaps some *anger* over a frustrating situation that just occurred, or *grief* stemming from a feeling of loss or a past trauma that has been triggered. Maybe I'm feeling bored (*apathy*), or nervous (*fear*) . . . whatever. If I stand by my reasons for these states, I am now identified with them and cannot see anything further. It will color everything I interpret and do. Perhaps I am seeking approval or a promotion at work (*desire*). Perhaps the session begins and is going well, so I think am an excellent music therapist (*pride*). Then things go bad. I am a lousy music therapist, in fact, a worthless human being (*grief*). My client is also dealing with the feelings of the day and the conceptions that accompany them, as well as a history that may well have established long-term patterns of *shame, guilt, apathy, grief, desire, anger*.

If I can be aware of all this internal evaluation, then it is my ethical responsibility to do what I can to move into higher states of consciousness. How do I do this? I've been in this position many times before. The training and experience that I've internalized to manage this situation connects me with states halfway up the scale right away, because I know I can tap into *willingness* and *courage* to deal with the circumstances, whatever they may be. I also know, from studying and believing Carl Rogers's (1961) concept, that unconditional *acceptance* of my client will activate the best chance of being effective. I continually look for feedback from my client. I will not respond emotionally or personally to any troubling behavior or negative feedback. I am a scientist, a truth-seeker, and have evoked *reason*. Although I can't say for sure how this process to raise my thought vibrations is going to translate directly to my client, I am doing my best to monitor my thought patterns and meet my client with my highest level of consciousness. Hopefully, the musical choices and forms of communication that stem from this intention will be received by the client in a positive manner.

Can I be a scientist as well as a musician? My clinician mind can stay with *reason* while my musician (as well as my client's musician) can access the higher realms. As music therapists, we have the extra, added, wonderful benefit of music to help in breaking away from the intellectual, as expressed by Hazrat Inayat Khan (1983):

> *What is wonderful about music is that it helps us to concentrate or mediate independently of thought and therefore music seems to be the bridge over the gulf between form and the formless. If there is anything intelligent, effective and at the same time formless, it is music.*

I can tap into some transpersonal assistance through my *willingness* to enter into my full, undivided presence through the *Creative Now* and my *intention* to move to higher states of consciousness to be of greatest service to my client. Hawkins (2006) asserts:

The combination of attention plus intention activates and accelerates the progression to higher levels of consciousness, and that the power of the higher levels of consciousness increases logarithmically. Thus, the influence of spiritual intention can be many times more powerful than ordinary intellectual effort.

EXPRESSION VS. DEPRESSION: SHIFTING THE DIRECTIONALITY OF LIFE ENERGY

While indulging in my lower states of consciousness may be ineffective for me as a clinician, all feelings as experienced or expressed by my client are acceptable in a therapy session. I cannot legitimately help to shift a client's vibrational state and its resultant interpretations, images, feelings, thoughts, and behaviors unless I allow them to be authentically expressed in the first place. In order to raise our state of consciousness, it is necessary to accept what is, fully and completely, exactly as we are and our client is, right now. However, it may be helpful to identify the directionality of the vibratory energy.

The words expression and depression have the same root: press, meaning an action of pressure or pushing, from Latin, *pressūra*: to urge, compel, force. In the case of those words, we are referring to life energy—emotions, intentions, will to survive. Express means to allow the life energy to flow; move in an outward direction. Depress means to reverse the natural outward flow of life energy; move it in an inward direction. Many people might say the opposite of depression is happiness, but based on this understanding: *The opposite of Depression is Expression.*

There are related words also built on the same root:

- *Repress*—to hold back the energy
- *Suppress*—to keep the energy down
- *Oppress*—to get in front of the energy so that it has nowhere to go before it even starts.

Repression, a well-known psychoanalytic term, can refer to an unconscious holding back of troubling feelings and thoughts from awareness. People can also be repressed, oppressed, or suppressed by forces from the outside, meaning other people.

When life energy becomes stuck or maladaptive, it needs awareness and resources to move it in a useful direction. Music has the power to do that, but a clinician must be willing to engage, rather than simply repress, oppress, or suppress, meaning be overly rigid, controlling, or censoring. As we attempt to nudge the client in the direction of higher states, we reach for the full range of "Clinical Musicianship," as Clive Robbins has explained it, that elusive blend of:

- Creative Freedom
- Intuition
- Expressive Spontaneity
- Right Musical Construction
- Clinical Responsibility

Here is a story by Clive Robbins that illustrates how this process can work:

We have a group class that comes in for the first session of the morning, and a boy who is usually very calm and cooperative is crying bitterly. And his teacher, rather elderly, has ten children to get ready for school, and this child has come in dirty because his mother had him take the garbage out to the sidewalk to put it in the can for collection. At the same time, the school bus was coming to pick this boy up, and the boy spilled the garbage on the sidewalk. And his mother made him pick it up with his hands. So he is dirty, he is in trouble, the bus has to wait for him for a moment, and the people are impatient. He gets on the bus, and the matron will not let him sit by anyone else, as he is dirty. So he is already crying by the time he gets to school. The teacher now has 10 of them to get ready for the first class, which is music, and she has to clean up the boy. So there is a terribly negative mood, and he is crying bitterly, and the teacher is impatient with him. Nordoff sees this from the piano and has an intuition. The intuition is, I can fix this with a song. So he improvises a song, very simple words:

"When you feel like crying, yes, when you feel like crying just cry, just cry."

It is a very slow, gentle and pentatonic melody. And the boy stops crying, and we have the class sing it, and the teacher sings it, and after ten minutes the whole bad mood is dissipated and we are in a good mood to start work. It is so simple, yet the intuition was there, and the melodic inspiration came in. So those are faculties we need, we depend on. We take intuition very seriously; it is a way of insight, a way of perception that we have to foster, and we encourage the development of these faculties in all our students.

THE TRANSCENDENCE OF INDIVIDUAL IDENTITY: THE WHOLE UNIVERSE IS SINGING

As Dr. Robbins's story illustrates, if we can make the right kind of music, even in response to states of *grief, shame, guilt, fear, anger,* or any type of uncomfortable state, the music may still bring us together—we may achieve an immersion in the "creative now" and we will be successful in the process of raising the client's state of consciousness.

> *Multiple experiences like this over time can shift a client's outlook permanently. That, in my view, is the essence of music therapy.*

We are the music, the music is us. The players become one in music. It is the loosening of the feeling of separateness that leads us to higher energy levels. According to Ken Wilber (1985), unity consciousness, in short, is nonboundary awareness. As the boundaries between us are diminished and ultimately revealed as the illusions they are, we move beyond individual identity. We are the same in heart and spirit. Perhaps we've conjured up feelings of *love.* "To see myself in everybody, and everybody in myself, most certainly is love," said Indian guru, Nisargadatta Maharaj (2000), who wrote the masterpiece of nondualistic thinking, *I Am That.*

Can our music, our joining in one creation, one sound, bring us into states of *joy* and *peace,* perhaps all the way up the scale to *enlightenment*? Explanations of *enlightenment* can vary. Is the experience attainable for mere mortals? According to Eckhart Tolle (2004), author of the best-selling book *The Power of Now,* absolutely:

> *The word enlightenment conjures up the idea of some superhuman accomplishment, and the ego likes to keep it that way, but it is simply your natural state of felt oneness with Being. It is a state of connectedness with something immeasurable and indestructible, something that, almost paradoxically, is essentially you and yet is much greater than you. It is finding your true nature beyond name and form.*

Based on Tolle's simple definition, I can say I've been to that place through music. Maybe I don't stay there but I have visited in the midst of a "Creative Now" moment. It's not an impossibly rare achievement. It is simply a glimpse of our true nature, and I am convinced music can bring us there. Sometimes clients will report experiences through music that parallel this definition of *enlightenment.* Unless I am told, I may not be able to comment definitively about a client's subjective experience; however, I certainly have observed noticeable shifts in affect that appear as deep immersion in the moment, *joy* and *peace,* as well as having experienced an uncanny unity in our collaborative music. This is the most marvelous experience, familiar to most musicians; a release from the loneliness of ego, as discussed by Dr. Ken Aigen (2005):

> *I would like to suggest that in the most powerful of musical experiences where there is a merging with the music or a transcendence of individual identity, something occurs that is like the river example. The specification of the nature of the experience in musical terms is no longer as relevant or even possible. One is in the music so completely that it disappears as an external entity, and its concrete parameters are not what is of the greatest relevance to the experiencer. Instead, it is the experience afforded by being the music that is most prominent. It may be more accurate to say that this is not an experience of music but an experience of oneself and the external world as music. (pp. 336–37)*

The music begins playing *through* you rather than being played *by* you; the "real YOU," as Alan Watts referred to it: The real deep down YOU is the Whole Universe; your living organism and all its behavior, it's expressing it as a singer sings a song. . . . You are something that the Whole Universe is doing, in the same way that a wave is something that the Whole Ocean is doing.

According to Bohm's concept of the Implicate Order, a part of the whole contains all the information of the whole, and changing a part of the whole changes the whole. The Attractor Patterns at the higher levels of consciousness we've placed into action—*Love, Peace, Joy, Enlightenment*—function not only as dynamic forces for healing in my client's life, as well as my own, but, as we have just discussed, they go forth and become available to bring healing for all who are willing to receive it.

> *Individual salvation actually has very little meaning, because, as I have pointed out, the consciousness of mankind is one and not truly divisible. Each person has a kind of responsibility not, however in the sense of answer-ability or guilt. But in the sense that there's nothing else to do, really, you see. There is no other way out. That is absolutely what has to be done and nothing else can work. —David Bohm (in Weber 1987)*

ROSE: SET THE ARTIST FREE

If there was a client I've known who consciously tried with all her might to access the higher levels of consciousness, it was Rose. She unceasingly studied literature, both contemporary and classic, relating to healing and spiritual wisdom. We would have long discussions about a wide range of spiritual topics: The Course in Miracles, the Akashic Records, the Tao te Ching, the Bible, angels, chakras, Buddha, Krishna, Jesus. She was hungry for it. But for Rose, ideas were not enough. As Jung (1967) said: "One does not become enlightened by imagining figures of light, but by making the darkness conscious" (p. 264). She did the best she could, but not many people have as much to transcend as did Rose.

Rose was a 43-year-old woman who had been a heroin user and prostitute most of her adult life. In addition to enduring a poverty-stricken childhood, she suffered relentless and terrible physical, emotional, and sexual abuse by her father. Rose was an extremely unstable woman whose mood swings, descents into depression, rage, identity confusion, impulsiveness, and possibly even occasional psychotic episodes suggested a borderline personality disorder.

She longed to be the embodiment of the self-realized individual she read about, but her dual existence as a spiritual seeker/junkie-prostitute was not so easily reconciled. She couldn't live inside her own skin. Neither persona could reconcile with the other, making her inner life barely tolerable. She did, in fact, have constant suicidal ideation and made several suicide attempts when she was younger.

Rose possessed a powerful artistic talent. She drew, painted, had a beautiful singing voice, and was able to improvise lyrics quite fluently. Of course, I was highly encouraging of Rose's first tentative efforts in music therapy, and through my support and her natural ability, Rose began to explore her inner world. Initially, she required two conditions for her creativity to emerge. First, the social environment had to be unconditionally supportive. If another member began to take a leadership role within the group, Rose would find a reason to leave. She was absolutely unable to face the slightest ego competition, though she raged about it internally. She would find me after the group fuming about some other person in the group who thought he was so great and was treating her like she was nothing. . . . In fact, this other person was just participating in the group the same as Rose, but she seemed to equate taking a supportive position with being intimidated and invisible.

Second, the music also had to be unconditionally supportive. She couldn't pay attention to chord changes, meter, or any demands the music might be making on her. Because of this, she was unable to stay with the accepted version of a popular song when she sang. Although we often sang songs, her interpretation was entirely idiosyncratic, and I would have to adjust my accompaniment moment-to-moment, as she would stretch out or rush her phrasing to suit her expressive inclinations of the moment. If other group members were attempting to sing or play along in a conventional way, she would invariably lose track of the rhythm and chord movement. Consequently, Rose's most successful musical accompaniment for her spontaneous improvisations was a one-chord repetitive drone. This music gave her absolute freedom and support.

The psychodynamic concept of the "shadow" is generally thought of as the hateful, angry, fearful aspects of the personality, too unacceptable to be consciously acknowledged, but psychodynamic music therapy pioneer Mary Priestly (1987) also discussed the modern Jungian concept of the "bright shadow," which contains unrealized positive potential. Carolyn Kenny (1982) also describes the relationship between music and the multidimensional shadow: "Shadow responds to music. It is the secret side, the quiet, hidden side. It can be the dark side we mask so easily—evil, fear, sorrow, pain. It can also be hidden joy and exuberance" (p. 90).

Rose's "bright shadow" emerged after approximately a year of me working with her. At the time, she claimed to be drug-free and attending Narcotics Anonymous meetings. In this session, a synthesizer was set up to vamp on a chord, while I accompanied on guitar and another group member played the conga. Nothing had been specifically planned, but what took shape was a song in a folk/rock/new-age style. Singing in her beautiful soprano voice, Rose improvised the following lyrics:

Set the Artist Free

Voices in my head criticize instead of letting go a song
Deeply within, it longs to sing a dream and dream a song
A universal melody that sets the artist free
Set the poet free

Feel the ocean breeze sweep across my soul
Telling stories not yet told
So bold, like a seagull's dive gently to the sea
It's about the artist in you and me seeking to be free
Yearning to be born
Yearning for the birth
A spiritual birth of chi and energy
That overrides the universal melody in you and me

Together as one we reach the higher act of speech
Exaggerated voice that turns inside our hand
A song is born to single

Upon a flight of birds
The peacock spreads its wings
Colorful feathers, a harmony, a unity comes together
It's you, it's true
It's new
Set the artist free
The poet is inside of me

In her poetic imagery, the sweep of her melody, the vibrato in her voice, Rose's song strives to manifest the beauty and artistry she seeks in herself and the world. The serene and pastoral one-chord harmonic bed produced by the synthesizer, my support, and the support of another client all helped to create the conditions that Rose needed in this session to make contact with her "bright shadow." Her well-realized conception and execution represented significant strengths. We recorded the piece on a multitrack recorder and overdubbed some additional background vocals and effects to further reinforce her connection with this positive part of herself.

Rose's dark shadow began to show itself in a music therapy session a few months later. In this session, to further experiment with the musical drone we had been exploring, we used the following musical setup: I had prepared a synthesizer by taping down one key in the lower register. While it played, I added modal chords on guitar with occasional arpeggios; one client played another open-chord-tuned guitar and another played various percussion instruments. Rose sang. This time, Rose's lyrical improvisations emerged out of music that took on a slow, dark, brooding quality:

He said do you want to sit and talk
Have a smoke and drink with me
I tell you, I was scared, so scared
This man—his eyes—so deep, so black
His heart—it had a hidden song for me

I thought of Dracula, a vampire
He seemed to want to take me on a flight this night
This tall man in a black cape with black gloves
Filled with hatred in his heart
He scared me

He said little girl, come away into the night with me
Come away, little girl
He said I've got a story to tell you of glory
Of high noon and bats and runes
And grey clouds and stormy weather
He said I've got a potion to give you if you've got a notion
To tell me which direction you aim to go in this evening

He read into my sad eyes
He knew I was so sad and despised
He knew I was confused

This tall man with his black cape
With his black hat
And his black velvety gloves
Didn't speak about love

He saw me crying beneath the willow
Quietly I wept in a secret fashion
As he approached the gate, he opened it and he'd state
Come away little girl
Come away with me,
Don't you see the end of the world is near

I'll take you to a place
Where you'll know the pain on your face
And the hatred you have in your heart
You'll become a part of the night
And you can release the screams in your mind
And you can swirl and turn and whirl and fall into a pit
Of gray and green and blue that seems like a dream
But it's really a nightmare
He said I'll take you away from here

Come away little girl
Come into the night little girl
Come away little girl, come away
Let me take you away . . .

As the music droned on ominously, the group spontaneously broke into the tortured screams of the damned. It was chilling. The lyrics Rose created illustrate her powerful fantasy life and romanticism of her own pain. Terrified, yet seduced, she is powerless to resist the evil influences calling to her. Herman (1992) reports that survivors of child abuse consistently have "overwhelming feelings of helplessness. . . . Unable to find any way to avert the abuse, they learn to adopt a position of complete surrender" (p. 98).

Unknown to me at the time, Rose had begun using heroin again. Maybe she never actually stopped, despite her claims to the contrary. The drugged, trancelike feel of the piece and Rose's resigned vocal delivery might be seen as a psychological regression from the previous piece, but it actually hits closer to the core of her pathology, and in that sense it represents a step forward. Although still disguised with the mythological theme, Rose is revealing a far more hidden aspect of her personality. The lyrics reflect her dark shadow in the form of Dracula, the archetypal demon-lover. Rose was very aware of the pernicious yet seductive trap of heroin. She is in control of her emotional projection, using her ambivalence in the face of annihilation to create an artistic statement. Our subsequent discussion of the piece's symbolism brought greater understanding to Rose's unconscious process. By embodying and giving voice to these conflicting aspects of herself, Rose began to bring consciousness to her intrapsychic battle.

A few months after this session, Rose was able to find some integration. She came into a music therapy session extremely upset by what she claimed to be a vicious rumor about her by her peers. Considering her psychological split, whatever people were saying about her might very well have been true, but that is beside the point. The music group that day consisted of Rose and, serendipitously, three other clients whom she trusted and who supported her. The intensity that Rose brought into the room inspired a driving drum improvisation, as Rose screamed out a verbal torrent of anger and pain in her improvised lyrics. This indicated meaningful progress, because in the prior two pieces, her defensiveness and self-involvement had prevented her from becoming fully involved. She was singing about herself or creating a fantasy using herself as a character, but she still maintained her distance and emotional control. In this session, she was totally present, channeling her rage in the creative now. She had previously not even attended sessions in her angry, chaotic moods, as she seemed to feel she needed to be in a calm, centered mood to make music. Now, she was truly sharing herself in the music, not just an idea about herself but the side of herself by which she felt extremely threatened. Jung proposed (1959) that the problem of the shadow is answered through relatedness. In the development of consciousness, we are gradually liberated from the imprisonment of unconsciousness. Mary Priestly (1987) relates this process to music therapy:

> *Music can express any emotion, conscious or unconscious. It can be the brittle music of self-defense, the shallow passing mood of the moment or a hauntingly deep voice from the shadow which may need a great deal of therapy before it is safely assimilated into the patient's consciousness. It takes training and experience to be aware of the seminal nature of these musical suggestions from the shadow, but when they are answered in the right moment and in the right way, radical healing can take place. (p. 26)*

I met with Rose some years after we stopped working together to ask for her consent to publish her song lyrics in an article I was writing (Soshensky, 2001). I had moved on to another professional position, and she was living the same lifestyle. She was pleased to have her story be told, but seemed sad and resigned to me. For a period, she was an artist, making music, painting pictures, having deep discussions about philosophical and spiritual principles. The part of her that was so far away from her street junkie/prostitute persona had a channel and permission to live.

Rose's life and mine had intersected in a profound way, and when we met that day two years later, we both knew she was going her way and I was going mine. Despite her deep aspirations to be a sober, working, reasonably emotionally healthy person with a hopeful future, she was stuck in a lifestyle and a pattern of behavior that was in deep opposition to that and from which she was unlikely to escape.

Rose was a brilliant, talented, spiritual, creative person, and it's not too hard to understand how a soul as passionate and sensitive as Rose could spiral out of control following the brutal treatment she received as a child. "There is strong shadow where there is much light," wrote Goethe (1773). Sometimes, maybe the length of the shadow, the unresolved pain and anger, the path one's life has taken under the force of its own momentum, is just too much to overcome.

Although organized religions, motivational speakers, and self-help authors are always trying to promote their point of view, there are no easy answers as to how people can overcome such difficult circumstances. Rose tried religion. She tried Narcotics Anonymous. She read all the books on spiritual healing she could get her hands on. Maybe these things work for some people. They didn't work for her. Her shame, guilt, anger, and other lower states of consciousness as identified by David Hawkins were too active, crushing, overpowering. "If there is meaning in life at all," wrote Viktor Frankl (1984), "then there must be meaning in suffering."

So what did it all mean? Did all that joyous creativity and soul-charged work amount to anything?

12

Curing versus Healing

So don't be frightened, dear friend, if a sadness confronts you larger than any you have ever known, casting its shadow over all you do. You must think that something is happening within you, and remember that life has not forgotten you; it holds you in its hand and will not let you fall. Why would you want to exclude from your life any uneasiness, any pain, any depression, since you don't know what work they are accomplishing within you?

—*Rainer Maria Rilke (in* Letters to a Young Poet*)*

A conventional way of thinking about psychotherapy, as defined on the Mayo Clinic website (www.mayoclinic.org), is that it helps you learn about your moods, feelings, thoughts, and behaviors, and it helps you learn how to take control of your life with healthy coping skills. I think that for many music therapists working with clients who have significant degrees of impairment, this characterization might require some reconsideration. I have worked with clients for whom such a definition may apply; people who still retained sufficient functional capabilities to have a chance for recovery and a better life—young people trying to reconcile traumatic childhoods or recover from acute mental health or addiction problems, middle-aged adults who have sustained significant challenges such as serious disease, injury, or stroke. I have worked with many more who have never had any real control over their lives and will never make it into the mainstream of typical activity. Or, if they were, at one time, in more mainstream activity with jobs, relationships, children, social lives, career, and personal aspirations, it is over. They will never make it back. People with severe chronic mental illness, Alzheimer's disease, terminal illness, nonverbal autism, chronic drug addiction and alcoholism, severe traumatic brain injury—the list goes on and on. How do we redefine therapy in this context?

Sometimes when there is little or no chance of changing the big picture, we can recognize a distinction between curing and healing. The word curing can represent a reductionist view, fragmenting a diagnosis from the whole person. If the presenting symptoms can be eliminated, the patient is considered to be cured or in remission. Healing has a broader connotation, encompassing the enhancement of emotional and spiritual components, as well. Moments of insight, acceptance, faith, connection, hope, and courage—these do not fade away. A person who might be incurable can still heal. Even if a person's death is imminent, healing is valuable, in and of itself.

David Bohm (1980) believed that in music, one is directly perceiving the Implicate Order, that is, the universal whole. Eminent music therapist, Dr. Kenneth Bruscia (2000), also felt that music provides experiences of ultimate meaningfulness through contact with the Implicate Order. Music locates, focuses, and expands our consciousness as it connects personal and transpersonal realms of experience. Dr. Bruscia asserts that the goal of therapy is to help the client find greater meaning. Through an interpersonal process of making meaning through music, we construct, deconstruct, and reconstruct our experiences of the Implicate Order so that they have meaning within our personal world. In his classic book, *Man's Search for Meaning*, Viktor Frankl (1984) wrote:

> *If there is meaning [in life], it is unconditional meaning, and neither suffering nor dying can detract from it. And what our patients need is unconditional faith in unconditional meaning. Remember what I have said of life's transitoriness. In the past, nothing is irrevocably lost but everything is irrevocably stored. People only see the stubble field of transitoriness but overlook the full granaries of the past in which they have delivered and deposited, in which they have saved their harvest. (p. 156)*

AKASHIC RECORDS: NOTHING IS IRREVOCABLY LOST, BUT EVERYTHING IS IRREVOCABLY STORED

> *As large as this Ether is, so large is that Ether within the heart. Both heaven and earth are contained within it, both fire and air, both sun and moon, both lightning and stars. . . .*
>
> —*Chandogya Upanishad, 8.1.3. (7th century, BC)*

What does Frankl (1984) mean when he says "nothing is irrevocably lost but everything is irrevocably stored"? He doesn't specifically refer to the life of the soul beyond the body, although during his experience of greatest torment in Auschwitz, he recalls these lines from Milton's *Paradise Lost*:

> *The angels are lost in perpetual*
> *contemplation of an infinite glory.*

He expands on this idea, writing that love goes beyond the physical person, finding its deepest meaning in the spiritual being of one's inner self. Whether or not one's beloved is actually present or even alive ceases to be of importance.

I don't know what Frankl's view was on a concept that has been called the Akashic Records. Amazingly, I first learned about this idea from Rose. She said, "You never heard about the Akashic Records, Rick? Well . . ." She was so happy to be teaching me. The Akashic Records, as Rose explained, were vibrational impressions, stored in the Etheric realm, of every deed, word, feeling, thought, and intent that has ever occurred throughout the history of the world, as well as a source for all future possibilities and every idea and evolution of consciousness yet to come. Therefore, in accordance with John Wheeler's *Participatory Anthropic Principle*: We are participants in bringing into being not only the near and here, but the far away and long ago.

According to this belief, the Akashic Records contain the underlying stimulus for every archetypal symbol, mythic story, or transformational invention that has shaped patterns of human behavior and experience. In the Sanskrit and Indian cultures, Akasha is an all-encompassing medium that underlies all things and becomes all things. It is real, but so subtle that it cannot be perceived until it becomes the many things that populate the manifest world (Laszlo, 2004). Hmmm . . . sounds a bit like quantum physics and, again, we see the concurrence of mysticism and contemporary science, as in Wheeler's statement, "No phenomenon is a real phenomenon until it is an observed phenomenon."

Although Akasha is a Sanskrit word, the Akashic Records, sometimes referred to as "The Book of Life," has been noted by Western writers, philosophers, and mystics, as well. There seems to be some relationship to Jung's concept of the Collective Unconscious, the shared archetypes, images, and memories of human experience that are passed down from generation to generation. There are related Bible passages, such as Psalm 56:8–9 (Revised Standard Version): "Thou hast kept count of my tossings; put thou my tears in thy bottle; are they not in thy book?"

The best-known contemporary Western source regarding the Akashic Records was the famous psychic, Edgar Cayce (Wyatt, 2014, p. 104), who said in one of his readings:

Upon time and space is written the thoughts, the deeds, the activities of an entity—as in relationships to its environs, its hereditary influence; as directed—or judgment drawn by or according to what the entity's ideal is. Hence, as it has been oft called, the record is God's book of remembrance; and each entity, each soul—as the activities of a single day of an entity in the material world—either makes same good or bad or indifferent, depending upon the entity's application of self towards that which is the ideal manner for the use of time, opportunity and the expression of that for which each soul enters a material manifestation. The interpretation then as drawn here is with the desire and hope that, in opening this for the entity, the experience may be one of helpfulness and hopefulness. (Reading 1650–1651)

An interesting point made in Cayce's statement above is that which determines the "goodness" or "badness" of a thought or deed is "the entity's application of self towards that which is the ideal manner for the use of time, opportunity and the expression of that for which each soul enters a material manifestation." As such, the Akashic Records guide, educate, and transform every individual to make the best use of his or her experience; each person writes the story of his or her life through thoughts, deeds, and involvement with the rest of creation. The Akashic Records encompass an ever-changing fluid array of possible futures that are called into the observable world as we interact with the data that has already been accumulated.

YOU ARE THE UNIVERSE

Stop acting so small. You are the universe in ecstatic motion. Everything in the universe is within you. Ask all from yourself.

—Rumi (1995)

Cayce's view of the mind, congruent with the view of modern physics, is that there is only one mind. Nobel Prize–winning Austrian physicist Erwin Schrodinger (1967) wrote:

I submit that both paradoxes will be solved . . . by assimilating into our Western build of science the Eastern doctrine of identity. Mind is by its very nature a singulare tantum. I should say: the over-all number of minds is just one. I venture to call it indestructible since it has a peculiar timetable, namely mind is always now. There is really no before and after for mind. There is only a now that includes memories and expectations. But I grant that our language is not adequate to express this, and I also grant, should anyone wish to state it, that I am now talking religion, not science.

Individual consciousness is like a tiny point coming out of the infinite consciousness, which connects to all superconscious and subconscious awareness. Clearly, many people would be skeptical about this idea—that any individual can access information from any location or source in the universe, including living or dead people, as well as sources of consciousness that have yet to be embodied.

Dr. Ken Aigen related this story about Clive Robbins following Robbins's passing (http://www.heerarajagopal.com/ow/dr-clive-robbins-1927-2011/):

One area in which Clive and I were quite different was in the area of esoteric and spiritual belief systems. He knew that I did not share his faith in phenomena such as reincarnation and communicating with extra-human spirits of various types, yet our mutual respect was so great that this area of difference did not diminish our relationship and affection for each other; it was something that we both acknowledged and that, in some ways, even enriched our relationship. Sometimes when you have fundamental differences with a person, it makes the areas of connection that much stronger.

So one day in the early 2000s, Clive walked into my office with a mixture of excitement, a mischievous glint in his eye, and about half a dozen copies of a book titled In the Spirit: Conversations with the Spirit of Jerry Garcia. *Clive was well aware of my strong affinity for Jerry Garcia, lead guitarist of the Grateful Dead. This book was written by Wendy Weir, the sister of Bob Weir, the rhythm guitarist of the band. The book recounted three years of conversations that the author reported having with the spirit of Jerry Garcia after his death in 1995. Clive liked to treat humorously what I knew he felt was my overly rational worldview that did not allow for the types of beliefs that were central to his own life. And I could see he was taking great pleasure in the fact that one of the touchstone figures in my life was now playing a central role in a drama concerning the world of the spirit.*

I was drawn to this book today as I was reflecting on what to write in this editorial. I opened the book and came to a page where the author poses a question to Garcia's spirit: "What message would you like to give?" Here is the reply:

One of love. I cannot say this enough. . . . Many of you have felt great pain and grief in my passing. This is a gift I have given you. Through the pain you have been able to search deeply within and release that love that radiates from your true self. You have reaffirmed your sense of self and sense of community. . . . The music is the vehicle for this love. Its energy, its vibration, breaks through the subtle barriers of human consciousness to free our inner selves, to give us the opportunity to discover who we truly are. (Weir, 1999, pp. 80–81)

DIE AND BE AGAIN

I don't think it would be any more unusual for me to show up in another life, than showing up in this one!

—*Eleanor Roosevelt (Dyer and Dyer, 2014)*

Do our sufferings, our mistakes, our regrets, our unfulfilled potentials, make more sense if viewed in the light of continuous learning on an immortal soul journey? "As long as you are not aware of the continual law of Die and Be Again, you are merely a vague guest on a dark Earth," said Goethe. David Hawkins (2006), whose ideas we have explored, believes that, like matter and energy, life cannot be destroyed. It can only change form. Thus, death is actually only the leaving of the body. The sense of identity is, however, unbroken. The state of "me" (self) is constant and continues after it separates from the physical expiration; that is, there has to be a "who" that goes on to another realm or chooses to reincarnate. And, as we traverse through this life, as Hawkins counseled, we try to maintain an awareness about which thought streams we aspire to dwell in most frequently. This is echoed in this (abridged by me) Tibetan Buddhist prayer to Chenrezeg, the pantheon of enlightened beings and embodiment of compassion:

I pray to you, my guru, Chenrezeg.
Buddha of great compassion, hold me fast in your compassion.
From time without beginning, beings have wandered in samsara,
Undergoing unendurable suffering.
Please bless them that they may achieve the omniscient state of buddhahood.

With the power of evil karma gathered from
beginningless time,
Sentient beings, through the force of anger, greed, stupidity, jealousy, pride
Are born as hell beings and experience
suffering.
May I, myself, through all my existences,
Act in the same manner as Chenrezeg.
By this means, may all beings be liberated
From the impure realms

The complete model of reincarnation, the one that agrees with all the reincarnational data, can now be stated proposes physicist, Dr. Goswami (2013):

> *Our various incarnations in the many different places and times are correlated beings, correlated by our intentions; information can transfer between these incarnations by virtue of the quantum non-local correlation. Behind the discreteness of the physical body and lived history of these incarnations, there exists a continuum; a continuum of the unfolding of meaning. Formally, the continuum is represented by the quantum monad (soul), a conglomerate of unchanging themes and changeable and evolving vital and mental propensities, or karmas. (p. 144)*

From another perspective, University of Arizona's Stuart Hameroff and British physicist Sir Roger Penrose claim they have found evidence of protein-based microtubules, structural components of human cells, that carry quantum information stored at a subatomic level. Penrose (2017) argues that when a person dies, this quantum information is released from the microtubules into the universe, and this quantum information can exist outside the body as what we might call soul. The body dies, but the spiritual quantum field continues.

NO AXE TO GRIND

I have no inside information. I'm not commenting on the rightness or wrongness of anyone's religious or spiritual beliefs. Nor am I saying I am clear about what happens beyond this mortal life of the senses. Like anyone, I read, learn, interact, live, and build my impressions about my life and work. As a music therapist, I've crossed paths with hundreds, maybe thousands, of people, none of whom were exactly living the good life. You've read about some profound connections with exceptional people; people who have contributed as much to me in my journey through this life as I have to them. With some clients, I can understand how I might have helped. For others, like Rose, what could I possibly do to counteract the severity of such a tragic life story? I have to take the long view—that, to repeat Cayce's words (Wyatt, 2014, p. 104): "The interpretation then as drawn here is with the desire and hope that, in opening this for the entity, the experience may be one of helpfulness and hopefulness."

That is my philosophical understanding—doing everything possible to discover and serve the creative purpose, not only of my client, but of the universe itself, regardless of how it seems to be going at the time or whether or not it appears to be successful treatment. Music therapy involves the discovery and manifestation of something new; the transformation of meaning; finding new meaning; the loosening of karmic patterns; being kind and respectful and attentive when maybe kindness and respect and attention are not expected.

CAN I CHANGE ALL THE DARKNESS AND MISERY IN THE WORLD? NO. CAN I BRING MUSIC INTO THOSE PLACES? YES.

I have been in some dark places in my music therapy career—institutions, programs, hospitals filled with masses of disenfranchised "patients" at the mercy of wheel-spinning, power-wielding bureaucrats and cynical practitioners; places with insufficient, misdirected, even misappropriated, funds, meant to serve people suffering from conditions, abuses, injuries, diseases, and struggles that no human being should have to contend with. They haven't all been like that. I've worked in more functional, conscientious places, too, and I certainly hope my Music Therapy Studio reflects a higher purpose. But, always, the strife and pain, the desperate longing for a glimpse of hope in the human condition is profound.

* * *

There is a living, breathing wholeness to all that exists. Past, present, and future are illusory. The fields of the finite and infinite are in constant communication, even though the only thing that we seem to be able to see, hear, touch, remember, and describe is the field of the finite. According to David Bohm (1980):

> *This field is basically that which is manifest, or tangible. The essential quality of the infinite, by contrast, is its subtlety, its intangibility. This quality is conveyed in the word spirit, whose root meaning is "wind, or breath." This suggests an invisible but pervasive energy, to which the manifest world of the finite responds. This energy, or spirit, infuses all living beings, and without it any organism must fall apart into its constituent elements. That which is truly alive in the living being is this energy of spirit, and this is never born and never dies.*

Ervin Laszlo (2004) in his book, *Science and The Akashic Field,* writes: "The universe is a memory-filled world of constant and enduring interconnection, a world where everything informs—acts on and interacts—with everything else. We should apprehend this remarkable world with our heart as well as with our intellect" (p. 125).

> *What makes us feel drawn to music is that our whole being is music: our mind and body, the nature in which we live, the nature which has made us, all that is beneath and around us, it is all music.*
>
> —*Hazrat Inyat Khan (1991)*

AND THAT'S ALL I HAVE TO SAY ABOUT THAT

Considered in this manner, music therapy has little to do with goals in the conventional sense. It has to do with raising our clients' vibrations; influencing their thoughts, feelings, and actions; changing their concept of who they are and the things of which they are capable. It has to do with helping them to experience themselves as valued members of the human family and, more than this, as infinite beings in an infinite creation on an infinite journey. There is no cause of anything. All our explanations, our reasons, our diagnoses, our theories, our goals, our resistances, our blaming: they are simply boxes. An infinite understanding means there is another box inside and another outside the box, never-ending. As quantum physics informs us, actually there are no boxes at all, just one unbroken wholeness. But if you want to make boxes, it's okay. You can look inside any box you want. Give it a name. Decide whether it is a good box or not. There is always another box, another reason, another cause, another way to look at it. When we share so completely and fully in music that these boxes of reasons and the disparity between our apparent separate identities disappear completely, these become the vital experiences that uplift and transform the consciousness of our client and his or her social network, as well as ourselves. Even the most humble of all, the most seemingly unsuccessful, inconsequential life journey can have as meaningful a part to play, if not more so, than the most powerful and rich business person, as Krishnamurti and Bohm (1999) explains:

> *The successful people are not the ones who are building a new world. To be a real revolutionary requires a complete change of heart and mind, and how few want to free themselves. One cuts the surface roots; but to cut the deep feeding roots of mediocrity, success, needs something more than words, methods, compulsions. There seem to be few, but they are the real builders—the rest labor in vain. One is everlastingly comparing oneself with another, with what one is, with what one should be, with someone who is more fortunate. This comparison really kills. Comparison is degrading, it perverts one's outlook. And on comparison one is brought up. All our education is based on it and so is our culture. So there is everlasting struggle*

to be something other than what one is. The understanding of what one is uncovers creativeness, but comparison breeds competitiveness, ruthlessness, ambition, which we think brings about progress. Progress has only led so far to more ruthless wars and misery than the world has ever known.

Superficial identities are not what matters. There is no hierarchy of functionality or importance. As our clients discover themselves, as they re-create themselves within the Music Therapy Studio, their efforts bear witness to the faith, the optimism, and the indomitability of the human spirit. The vibratory impressions from which we draw our true identities that may have been entrenched in shame, apathy, grief, anxiety, anger, loneliness, and disease can become transformed into the realization of harmony, love, unity, joy, peace, hope, and happiness. In this metamorphosis, those who might otherwise be marginalized project their presence, their voices, their music proudly into the world as they offer their contribution to humanity's collective evolution toward higher states of consciousness.

References

Aasgaard, T. (2000). "A suspiciously cheerful lady." A study of a song's life in the pediatric oncology ward, and beyond. *British Journal of Music Therapy, 14*(2), 70–82.

Aasgaard, T. (2002). *Song creations by children with cancer: Process and meaning.* (Unpublished doctoral dissertation). Department of Music and Music Therapy, Aalborg University.

Abberly, P. (1987). The concept of oppression and the development of a social theory of disability. *Disability, handicap & society, 2*(1), 5–19.

Adam, D. (2013). Mental health: On the spectrum. *Nature, 496*: 7446. https://www.nature.com/news/mental-health-on-the-spectrum-1.12842.

Aigen, K. (1991). The voice in the forest: A conception of music for music therapy. *Music therapy, 10*(1), 77–98.

Aigen, K. (1993). The music therapist as qualitative researcher. *Music Therapy, 12*(1), 16–39.

Aigen, K. (1995). An aesthetic foundation of music therapy: An underlying basis for creative music therapy. In C. Kenny (Ed.), *Listening, playing, creating: Essays on the power of sound* (pp. 233–258). Albany, NY: State University of New York Press.

Aigen, K. (1996). *Being in music: Foundations of Nordoff-Robbins music therapy.* St. Louis, MO: MMB Music.

Aigen, K. (1998). *Paths of development in Nordoff-Robbins music therapy.* Gilsum, NH: Barcelona Publishing.

Aigen, K. (2001). Popular music styles in Nordoff and Robbins clinical improvisation. *Music therapy perspectives, 19* (1), 31–44.

Aigen, K. (2004). Conversations on creating community: Performance as music therapy in New York City. In M. Pavlicevic & G. Ansdell (Eds.), *Community music therapy* (pp. 186–213). London: Jessica Kingsley Publishers.

Aigen, K. (2005). *Music-centered music therapy*. Gilsum, NH: Barcelona Publishers LLC.

Aigen, K. (2014). Music-centered dimensions of Nordoff-Robbins music therapy. *Music Therapy Perspectives, 32*(1), 18–29.

Aigen, K. (2015). *Contemporary Social Movements in the Autism Community*. Lecture: Implications for Music Therapy Research. The Rebecca Center for Music Therapy at Molloy College Presents: International Perspectives on Improvisational Music Therapy and Autism Spectrum Disorder: Research and Practice; Friday, October 30, 2015.

Alcoholics Anonymous (1952), *Twelve steps and twelve traditions*, New York, NY: Alcoholics Anonymous World Services, Inc.

Aldridge, D. (2006). *Music therapy and neurological rehabilitation: Performing health*. London: Jessica Kingsley Publishers.

American Music Therapy Association website. https://www.musictherapy.org/.

AMTA Member Sourcebook. (2006). Silver Spring, MD: American Music Therapy Association.

Ananthaswamy, A. (2018). *Through two doors at once: The elegant experiment that captures the enigma of our quantum reality*. New York, NY: Dutton.

Ansdell, G. (1995). *Music for life: Aspects of creative music therapy with adult clients* (Vol. 1). London: Jessica Kingsley Publishers.

Ansdell, G. (2002). Community music therapy and the winds of change—a discussion paper. In C. Kenny & B. Stige (Eds.), *Contemporary voices in music therapy: Communication, culture and community* (pp. 109–143). Oslo, Norway: Unipub Forlag.

Ansdell, G. (2005). Being who you aren't; Doing what you can't: Community music therapy & the paradoxes of performance. *Voices: A World Forum for Music Therapy, 5*(3). Retrieved from https://doi.org/10.15845/voices.v5i3.229.

Aspect, A. (15 October 1976). "Proposed experiment to test the nonseparability of quantum mechanics." *Physical Review D. 14* (8): 1944–1951.

Austin, D. (2003). *When words sing and music speaks: A qualitative study of in-depth music psychotherapy with adults*. (Doctoral dissertation). New York University.

Austin, D., & Dvorkin, J. (1998). Resistance in individual music therapy. In K. Bruscia (Ed.), *The dynamics of music psychotherapy*. Gilsum, NH: Barcelona Publishers LLC.

Autistic Self Advocacy Network. Retrieved October 24, 2017, from http://autistic advocacy.org/.

Bailey, D. (1992). *Improvisation: Its nature and practice in music*. Cambridge, MA: DaCapo Press.

Bakan, M. (2018). Interview in *U.S. News and World Report*. Retrieved from https://www.usnews.com/news/the-report/articles/2018-06-08/music-is-a-powerful-tool-for-people-with-autism.

Baniel, A. (2012). *Kids beyond limits*. New York, NY: Perigee Books.

Barnes, C., & Mercer, G. (1996). Exploring the divide: Illness and disability. Leeds, UK: Disability Press.

Basch, M. F. (1988). *Understanding psychotherapy: The science behind the art*. New York, NY: Basic Books.

Bell, J. S., & Aspect, A. (2004). Speakable and unspeakable in quantum mechanics. In series, *Collected papers on quantum philosophy*. Cambridge, UK: Cambridge University Press.

Benzon, W. (2001). *Beethoven's anvil: Music in mind and culture*. New York, NY: Basic Books.

Bernstein, L. (2004). *The joy of music*. Cambridge, UK: Amadeus Press.

Bohm, D. (1980). *Wholeness and the implicate order*. London, UK, and New York, NY: Routledge.

Bosco, F. (1992). *Elemental music massage: An energy-based approach combining music and bodywork*. (Unpublished master's thesis). New York University.

Bowlby, J., & Parker, C. M. (1970). Separation and loss within the family. In E. Anthony & C. Koupernik (Eds.), *The child in his family (Vol. 1)*. New York, NY: John Wiley and Sons.

Bragg, M. (2007). The last remaining avant-garde movement. *Society Guardian*, December 11. www.guardian.co.uk.

Brendtro, L., Brokenleg, M., & Van Bockern, S. (1990). *Reclaiming youth at risk: Our hope for the future*. Bloomington, IN: Solution Tree Press.

Brown, S. (2001). Are music and language homologues? *Annals of the New York Academy of Sciences: The biological foundations of music, 930*, 372–374.

Browning, R. (1871). *Balaustion's adventure*. Boston: J.R. Osgood and Company.

Bruscia, K. (1995). Modes of conscience in guided imagery and music (GIM): A therapist's experience of the guiding process. In C. Kenny (Ed.), *Listening, playing, creating: Essays on the power of sound* (pp. 165–198). Albany, NY: State University of New York Press.

Bruscia, K. (1998). An introduction to music psychotherapy. In K. Bruscia (Ed.), *The Dynamics of music therapy*. Gilsum, NH: Barcelona Press.

Bruscia, K. (2000). The Nature of Meaning in Music Therapy. July 2000. *Nordic Journal of Music Therapy 9* (2): 84–96. DOI: 10.1080/08098130009478005

Bruscia, K. (2012). Ways of thinking in music therapy. https://www.musictherapy.org/new_amta-pro_podcast_featuring_dr_kenneth_e_bruscia/.

Campbell, E. M., & McMahon, P. A. (1976), *Please touch*. New York, NY: Sheed and Ward.

Campbell, J. (1949). *The hero with a thousand faces*. Princeton, NJ: Princeton University Press.

Carpente, J. (2013). *The individual music-centered assessment profile for neurodevelopmental disorders: A clinical manual*. Philadelphia, PA: Regina Publishers.

Carpente, John A. (2018). Goal Attainment Scaling: A method for evaluating progress toward developmentally based music-centered treatment goals for children with autism spectrum disorder. *Music Therapy Perspectives*, 36 (2), 2018. 215–223.

Carpente, J., & Aigen, K. (2019). A music-centered perspective on music therapy assessment. D. J. Elliott, M. Silverman, & G. E. McPherson (Eds.), *The Oxford handbook of philosophical and qualitative assessment in music education* (p. 249). New York, NY: Oxford University Press.

Carpente, J., & Gattino, G. (2018). Inter-rater reliability on the Individual Music-Centered Assessment Profile for Neurodevelopmental Disorders (IMCAP-ND) for autism spectrum disorder. *Nordic Journal of Music Therapy, 27* (4), 297–311.

Chalmers, D., & Koch, C. (2017). Will it ever be possible to measure subjective experience? *Massive Science*. Retrieved from https://massivesci.com/articles/will-it-ever-be-possible-to-measure-subjective-experience/.

Chandogya Upanishad (English Translation) by Swami Lokeswarananda. Roseville, MN: Ramakrishna Mission Institute of Culture. ISBN: 9788185843919

Cohen, L. (2015). Cohencentric: Leonard Cohen considered. https://cohencentric.com/2015/12/16/three-characteristics-that-make-a-song-a-leonard-cohen-song-3-artistic-design-the-mystery-practicality-of-songs/.

Coltrane, J. Retrieved from https://www.azquotes.com/author/3149-John_Coltrane.

Condeluci, A., & McMorrow, M. (2004). Philosophy of rehabilitation. In *Certification Exam Preparation Course*. American Academy for the Certification of Brain Injury Specialists.

Corker, C., & Shakespeare, T. (Eds.). (2002). *Disability/postmodernity: Embodying disability theory*. London: Continuum.

A Course in Miracles. (1975). Mill Valley, CA: Foundation for Inner Peace.

Cross, I. (1999). Is music the most important thing we ever did? Music, development and evolution. In S. Won Yi (Ed.), *Music, mind and science*. Seoul, Korea: Seoul National University Press.

Crowe, B. (2004). *Music and soulmaking: Toward a new theory of music therapy*. Lanham, MD: Scarecrow Press.

Csíkszentmihályi, M. (1988). *Optimal experience: Psychological studies of flow*. Cambridge: Cambridge University Press.

Csíkszentmihályi, M. (1990). *Flow: The psychology of optimal experience*. New York, NY: Harper and Row.

Csíkszentmihályi, M. (1999). *The systems model of creativity: The collected works of Mihaly Csikszentmihalyi*. Heidelberg, Germany: Springer Netherlands Publishing.

Daily Mail (2019). A blast of heavy metal "boosts blooms." Thursday, October 24, 2019. https://www.dailymail.com.uk/news/article-2311386/Study-Plants-listened-Black-Sabbath-best-flowers-listened-Cliff-Richard-died.html.

Daramola, I. (2018). The best, worst, and funniest moments from Jay-Z's interview with David Letterman. *Spin Magazine*, April 6, 2018. https://www.spin.com/2018/04/jay-z-david-letterman-interview-best-moments/.

Davies, R. (1970). Q&A: Afternoon tea with Ray Davies. *Rolling Stone Magazine*, November 26, 1970. Retrieved from https://www.rollingstone.com/music/music-news/qa-afternoon-tea-with-ray-davies-161322/.

Dewey, J. (1934). *Art as experience*. New York, NY: Wideview/Perigee.

Diamond, S. (2012). Why we love music—and Freud despised it. *Psychology today*. Retrieved from https://www.psychologytoday.com/ca/blog/evil-deeds/201211/why-we-love-music-and-freud-despised-it?amp.

Diener, E., Sapyta, J., & Suh, E. (1998). Subjective well-being is essential to well-being. *Psychological Inquiry*, *9*(1).

Dileo, C. (2000). *Ethical thinking in music therapy*. Cherry Hill, NJ: Jeffrey Books.

Dileo, C., & Bradt, J. (2005). *Medical music therapy: A meta-analysis and agenda for future research*. Cherry Hill, NJ: Jeffrey Books.

Dissanaake, E. (2014). The artful species engages in art behaviours. Commentary on Stephen Davies, *The Artful Species. Estetika: Central European Journal of Aesthetics* 7(1): 101–104.

Dixon, P. L. (1984). *The Olympian*. Santa Monica, CA: Roundtable Publishers.

Doyle, A. C. (1993). *The return of Sherlock Holmes*. London, UK: Oxford University Press.

Dubuffet, J. (1986). *Asphyxiating culture and other writings*. New York, NY: Four Walls Eight Windows.

Dyer, S., & Dyer, W. (2014). *Don't die with your music still in you*. Carlsbad, CA: HayHouse.

Dylan, B. (2012). Bob Dylan: The Paul Zollo Interview. *American songwriter*. https://americansongwriter.com/2012/01/bob-dylan-the-paul-zollo-interview-3/7/.

Einstein, A. (n.d.). A letter from Albert Einstein to his daughter: On the universal force of love. Retrieved from https://monoset.com/blogs/journal/a-letter-from-albert-einstein-to-his-daughter-on-the-universal-force-of-love.

Emerson, R. W. (2010). *The later lectures of Ralph Waldo Emerson, 1843–1871*, p. 340. Athens, GA: University of Georgia Press.

Erdrich, L. (2005). *The painted drum*. New York, NY: Harper Collins.

Erikson, E. H. (1963). *Childhood and society*. New York, NY: Norton.

Feinstein, D. (1979). Personal mythology as a paradigm for a holistic public psychology. *American Journal of Orthopsychiatry, 49* (2): 198–217.

Folger, T. (2002). Does the universe exist if we're not looking? *Discover Magazine*. June 1, 2002.

Frankl, V. (1984). *Man's search for meaning*. New York, NY: Simon and Schuster.

Fronsdal, G. (2005). *The Dhammapada: A new translation of the Buddhist classic*. Boston, MA: Shambhala Publications.

Gage, F. (2004). Structural plasticity of the adult brain. *Dialogues Clin Neurosci, 6*(2): 135–141.

Gardner, H. (1983), *Frames of mind: The theory of multiple intelligences*. New York, NY: Basic Books.

Gibran, K. (2009). *The treasured writings of Kahlil Gibran*. Edison, NJ: Castile Books.

Gitler, Ira. (1958). Trane on the track. *Down Beat*. Archived from the original on 2007-09-30. Retrieved 2008-02-15.

Goethe, J. (1773). *Götz von Berlichingen*, Act 1.

Goethe, J. (1824). *Wilhelm Meister's Apprenticeship*. (Trans. from the German by T. Carlyle.). London, UK: Chapman and Hall. p. 194.

Goldstein, E. B. (2010). *Encyclopedia of perception*. SAGE Publications. p. 492.

Gonzalez, D. (1992). *Mythopoetic music therapy: A phenomenological investigation into its application with adults*. (Unpuplished doctoral thesis). https://steinhardt.nyu.edu/scmsAdmin/media/users/jts390/Dissertations/Gonzalez_David_1992.pdf.

Gosling, J. Retrieved from http://www.ju90.co.uk/.

Goswami, A. (2013). *Physics of the soul: The quantum book of living, dying, reincarnation and immortality*. Charlottesville, VA: Hampton Roads Publishing Company.

Grandin, T. (2011). *The way I see it: A personal look at autism and Asperger's* (Revised and Expanded 2nd Edition). Arlington, TX. Future Horizons.

Hadley, S., & Norris, M. (2016). Musical multicultural competency in music therapy: The first step. *Music Therapy Perspectives, 34* (2), 129–137.

Hanser, S. (1999). *The new music therapist's handbook.* Boston, MA: Berklee Press.

Harburg, Y. Retrieved from http://yipharburg.com/.

Harrison, David (2002). *Complementarity and the Copenhagen interpretation of quantum mechanics.* Undergraduate physics students computing and learning environment department of physics University of Toronto. https://faraday.physics.utoronto.ca/.

Harvey, A. (2017). *Music, evolution, and the harmony of souls.* Oxford, UK: Oxford University Press. p. 167.

Hawkins, D. (1995). *Power vs. force: The hidden determinants of human behavior.* Carlsbad, CA: Hay House.

Hawkins, D. (2001). *The eye of the I (from which nothing is hidden).* Carlsbad, CA: Hay House.

Hawkins, D. (2006). *Transcending the levels of consciousness: The stairway to enlightenment.* Sedona, AZ: Veritas Publishing.

Heath, S. (2008). Let the music heal your soul. *Ulster Publishing's Guide to Mid-Hudson Health Services,* 2008–2009 edition.

Hemachandra, R. (2015). Ray Hemachandra@Golden Moon Circles. Living on a rampage of appreciation—An interview with Wayne Dyer. https://rayhemachandra.com/2020/05/25/wayne-dyer-interview1/.

Henry, R. C. (2005). The mental universe. *Nature, 436,* 29.

Herman, J. (1992). *Trauma and recovery: The aftermath of violence—from domestic abuse to political terror.* New York: Basic Books.

Hicks, S. (2014). *Beethoven on the metaphysics of music.* Retrieved from: https://www.stephenhicks.org/2014/01/31/beethoven-on-the-metaphysics-of-music/.

Holzman, L. (1999). *Performing psychology: A postmodern culture of the mind.* London: Routledge.

Homans, G. C. (1941). Anxiety and ritual: The theories of Malinowski and Radcliffe-Brown. *American Anthropologist;* New Series, *43* (2), Part 1 (April–June), 164–172.

Howlin, P., Goode, S., Hutton, J., & Rutter, M. (2004). Adult outcome for children with autism. *Journal of child psychology and psychiatry, 45*(2), 212–229.

Hunt, P. (1966). *Stigma: The experience of disability.* London: Geoffrey Chapman.

Hurt, C., Rice, R., McIntosh, G., & Thaut, M. (1998). Rhythmic auditory stimulation in gait training for patients with traumatic brain injury. *Journal of Music Therapy, 35*(4), 228–241.

Isaacson, W. (2007). *Einstein: His life and universe.* New York, NY: Simon and Schuster Paperbacks.

James, J. (1993). *The music of the spheres.* New York, NY: Copernicus.

James, W. (1901). *The varieties of religious experience: A study in human nature.* London: Longmans, Green and Co.

Jarrett K. (2009) Interview with Keith Jarrett. https://ethaniverson.com/interviews/interview-with-keith-jarrett/.

Jaynes, J. (1976). *The origin of consciousness in the breakdown of the bicameral mind.* Boston: Houghton Mifflin.

Jimi Hendrix Quotes. (n.d.). BrainyQuote.com. Retrieved October 9, 2018, from BrainyQuote.com Web site: https://www.brainyquote.com/quotes/jimi_hendrix_195416.

John Coltrane Quotes. (n.d.). BrainyQuote.com. Retrieved October 9, 2018, from BrainyQuote.com Web site: https://www.brainyquote.com/quotes/john_coltrane_600683.

Johnson, G. (2018, February 26). Life in the trauma vortex. *Spiritual Psychology*. https://issp.inner-growth.org/life-in-the-trauma-vortex/.

Joplin, K., & Dvorak, A. (2016). A survey exploring the current state of censorship in adult psychiatric music therapy practice. *Music Therapy Perspectives, 35* (2, 13): 199–208.

Josephson, B., & Pallikari, F. (1991). Biological utilisation of quantum non-locality. *Foundations of Physics* (Vol. 21), pp. 197–207, (c) Plenum Press.

Jung, C. G. (1938). *Psychology and religion: West and east*. New York, NY: Routledge.

Jung, C. G. (1959). *Collected works of C.G. Jung, Volume 9 (Part 1): Archetypes and the collective unconscious*. G. Adler (Ed.). Princeton, NJ: Princeton University Press.

Jung, C. G. (1967). *The collected works of C. G. Jung (Vol. 13)*. G. Adler (Ed.). Princeton, NJ: Princeton University Press.

Jung, C. G. (1969). *Archetype and the collective unconscious*. Princeton, NY: Princeton University Press.

Jung, C. G. (1973). *Letters of C. G. Jung: Volume I, 1906–1950*. G. Adler, & A. Jaffe (Eds.). Abingdon, UK: Taylor and Francis.

Kaplan, S. (2002). *Different paths, different summits: A Model for religious pluralism*. Lanham, MD: Rowman and Littlefield Publishers, Inc.

Keats, J. (2004). *Ode on a Grecian urn and other poems*. Whitefish, MT: Kessinger Publishing.

Keenen, G. (2002). *Liner notes for do I dare?* New York, NY: Gardenia Productions.

Kenny, C. (1982). *The mythic artery*. Atascadaro, CA: Ridgeview Publishing.

Kenny, C. (1989). *The field of play*. Atascadaro, CA: Ridgeview Publishing.

Kenny, C. (2002). Keeping the world in balance: Music therapy in a ritual context. *Voices: A World Forum for Music Therapy*, 7 (1). https://voices.no/index.php/voices/article/view/1591.

Khan, H. I. (1962). *Spiritual development by the aid of music. The Sufi message of Hazrat Inayat Khan*, II. Geneva, Switzerland: Wassenaar Publications.

Khan, H. I. (1991). *The mysticism of sound and music: The Sufi Teaching of Hazrat Inayat Khan*. Boston, MA: Shambhala Publications.

Khan, H. I. (1993). *The music of life*. New York, NY: Omega Publications, p. 134.

Khan, H. I. (2011). *The way of illumination: The Sufi message: Volume One*. Motilal Banarsidass Publishers Pvt. Ltd.

Khun, T. (1962). *The structure of scientific revolution*. Chicago: University of Chicago Press.

King, S. (1997). *Rituals and modern society*. Retrieved from https://www.huna.org/html/skritual.html.

Kissel, H. (2000). *Stella Adler: The Art of Acting*. New York, NY: Applause Books.

Klein, M. (1938). The Psychogenesis of manic-depressive states. *International Journal of Psychoanalysis, 16*, 145–175.

Klein, S. (2006). *The science of happiness: How our brains make us happy*. New York, NY: DeCapo Press.
Krishnamurti, J. (1992). *The collected works of J. Krishnamurti*, (1963–1964). The New Mind. Volume 14. Dubuque, IA: Kendall/Hunt.
Krishnamurti, J., & Bohm, D. (1999). *The limits of thought: Discussions between J. Krishnamurti and David Bohm*. London, UK: Routledge.
Kuppers, P. (2011). *Disability, culture and community performance: Find a strange and twisted shape*. Houndmills and New York, NY: Palgrave.
Lanza, R., & Berman, B. (2010). *Biocentrism: How life and consciousness are the keys to understanding the true nature of the universe*. Dallas, TX: BenBella Books.
Lao Tzu. (1988). *Tao te ching*. (Trans. S. Mitchell). New York, NY: Harper Collins.
Laszlo, E. (2004). *Science and the akashic field: An integral theory of everything*. Rochester, VT: Inner Traditions.
Levitan, D. (2006). *This is your brain on music: The science of a human obsession*. New York, NY: Plume.
Limb, C. (2008). *This is your brain on jazz: Researchers use MRI to study spontaneity, creativity*. https://www.hopkinsmedicine.org/news/media/releases/this_is_your_brain_on_jazz_researchers_use_mri_to_study_spontaneity_creativity.
Limb, C. (2017). What makes a genius? *National Geographic*. https://www.nationalgeographic.com/magazine/2017/05/genius-genetics-intelligence-neuroscience-creativity-einstein/.
Logis, M. Retrieved from http://www.marialogis.com/story.
Longaker, C. (2003). Listening with presence, awareness and love. In M. Brady (Ed.), *The wisdom of listening* (p. 5). Somerville, MA: Wisdom Publications.
Lowen, A. (1975). *Bioenergetics*. New York, NY: Penguin Books.
Lowen, A. (2003). *Fear of life*. Hinesburg, VT: Alexander Lowen Foundation.
Lowey, J. (2000). Music psychotherapy assessment. *Music Therapy Perspectives, 18*(1), 47–58.
Magaret, A. (1950). Generalization in successful psychotherapy. *Journal of Consulting Psychology, 14*(1), 64–70. Retrieved September 14, 2017 from http://dx.doi.org/10.1037/h0053633.
Malik, K. (2017). In defense of cultural appropriation. *New York Times*. https://www.nytimes.com/2017/06/14/opinion/in-defense-of-cultural-appropriation.html.
Manning, A. G. et al. (2015). Wheeler's delayed-choice gedanken experiment with a single atom. *Nature physics*. doi: 10.1038/nphys3343
Marcus, J. (1995). The silent source. In C. Kenny (Ed.), *Listening, playing, creating: Essays on the power of sound*. Albany, NY: State University of New York Press.
Martino, P. http://www.patmartino.com/.
Maslach, C., & Goldberg, J. (1998). Prevention of burnout: New perspectives. *Applied and preventive psychology, 7*, 63–74.
Maslow, A. (1968). *Toward a psychology of being* (2nd ed.). New York, NY: Van Nostrand.
Maslow, A. (1987). *Motivation and personality* (3rd ed.). New York, NY: Harper and Row Publishers, Inc.
Matloff, G. (2016). Can panpsychism become an observational science? *Journal of Consciousness Exploration & Research, 7*, 7.

Matson, J. L, Benavidez, D. A, Compton, L. S, Paclawskyj, T., & Baglio, C. (1996). Behavioral treatment of autistic persons: A review of research from 1980 to the present. *Research in Developmental Disabilities, 17*, 433–465.
May, R. (1994). *The courage to create.* New York, NY: Norton. First published in 1975.
Mayo Clinic. Retrieved from https://www.mayoclinic.org.
Menon, V., & Levitin, P. (2005). The rewards of music listening: Response and physiological connectivity of the mesolimbic system. *NeuroImage, 28*(1), 175–184.
Merali, Z. (2015). Quantum "spookiness" passes toughest test yet. *Nature: International Journal of Science, 525*, 7567.
Merriam-Webster's collegiate dictionary. Retrieved from https://www.merriam-webster.com/.
Miller, G. F. (2000). *Evolution of human music through sexual selection.* In N. L. Wallin, B. Merker, & S. Brown (Eds.), *The origins of music* (pp. 329–360). Cambridge, MA: MIT Press.
Neumann, E. (1959). *Art and the creative unconscious.* Princeton, NJ: Princeton University Press.
Nguyenly, M. (2019, March 30). Woman faces dread of cancer with music therapy, finds healing and hope. *The Epoch Times.* https://www.theepochtimes.com/woman-faces-cancer-with-music-therapy-finds-healing-and-hope_2836055.html?fbclid=IwAR1kjwLu9YBhRilzm8VhatMehzch0mODK4mV7XjEH6jimUO-ZYnNTP0T_MU.
Nietzsche, F. (1999). *Thus spake Zarathustra.* New York, NY: Dover.
Nisargadatta Maharaj (2000). *I am that: Talks with Sri Nisargadatta Maharaj.* Charlottetown, Prince Edward Island, CAN: Acorn Press.
Nordoff, P. (1998). *Healing heritage: Paul Nordoff exploring the tonal language of music* (Clive Robbins and Carol Robbins, Eds.). Gisum, NH: Barcelona.
Nordoff, P., & Robbins, C. (1977). *Creative music therapy.* New York, NY: The John Day Company.
Nordoff, P., & Robbins, C. (2005). *Therapy in music for handicapped children* (reissue). Gilsum, NH: Barcelona Publishers LLC.
Nordoff-Robbins Center for Music Therapy website, https://steinhardt.nyu.edu/nordoff/the-practice/history#:~:text=Fellowship%20for%20music.-,Dr.,clinical%20use%20of%20improvised%20music
Oliver, M. (1992). Changing the social relations of research production. *Disability, handicap and society, 7*(2), 101–114.
Parker, C. Charlie Parker Quotes. (n.d.). BrainyQuote.com. Retrieved October 8, 2018, from BrainyQuote.com Web site: https://www.brainyquote.com/quotes/charlie_parker_400574
Parker, W. R. (1957). *Prayer can change your life.* New York, NY: Prentice-Hall.
Pavlicevic, M., & Ansdell, G. (Eds.). (2005). *Community music therapy.* London: Jessica Kingsley Publishers.
Peck, M. S. (1978). *The road less traveled: A new psychology of love, traditional values, and spiritual growth.* New York, NY: Simon and Schuster.
Pelias, R. (2004). *A methodology of the heart: Evoking academic and daily life.* Lanham, MD: Alta Mira Press.
Penrose, R. (1989). *The emperor's new mind.* Oxford, UK: Oxford University Press.

Penrose, R. (2017). Life after death? –Physicists says it's quantum information that transcends from one world to another. https://dailygalaxy.com/2017/08/life-after-death-renowned-physicists-says-its-quantum-information-stored-at-a-sub-atomic-level-that/.

Pines, A. M., & Keinan, G. (2005). Stress and burnout: The significant difference. *Personality and individual differences, 39*(3), 625–635.

Pinker, S. (1997). *How the mind works.* New York, NY: W.W. Norton.

Porges, S. (2011). *The polyvagal theory: Neurophysiological foundations of emotions, attachment, communication, and self-regulation.* New York, NY: W.W. Norton and Company.

Priestly, M. (1987). Music and the shadow. *Music Therapy,* 2(1), 20–27.

Pugatch, J. (2006). *Acting is a job: Real life lessons about the acting business.* New York, NY: Alworth Press.

Rea, S. (2015). Training by repetition actually prevents learning for those with autism. Retrieved October 19, 2017 from http://ww.cmu.edu/news/stories/archives/2015/october/repetition-and-autism.html.

Reisner, R. (1977) *Bird: The legend of Charlie Parker.* Boston, MA: DaCapo Press.

Rilke, R. M. (2000). *Letters to a young poet.* Novato, CA: New World Library.

Robbins, C., & Ritholz, M. (1999). Themes for therapy. In *Simon's Bells* by Sorel, S. New York, NY: Carl Fischer Music Publisher.

Robbins, C., & Robbins, C. (Eds.). (1998). *Healing heritage: Paul Nordoff exploring the tonal language of music.* Gilsum, NH: Barcelona Publishers LLC.

Rogers, C. R. (1961). *On becoming a person: A therapist's view of psychotherapy.* London: Constable.

Rogers, C. R. (1995). *A way of being.* Boston, MA: Mariner Books.

Rolvsjord, R. (2010). *Resource-oriented music therapy in mental health care.* Gilsum, NH: Barcelona Publishers LLC.

Rolvsjord, R. (2015). Resource-oriented perspectives in music therapy. *The Oxford Handbook of Music Therapy.* Jane Edwards (Ed.). Print Publication Date: Jan 2016. Online Publication Date: Jun 2015. doi: 10.1093/oxfordhb/9780199639755.013.5.

Rumi. (1995). *The essential Rumi.* Translation by C. Barks. New York, NY: Harper Collins.

Ruud, E. (1995). Improvisation as a liminal experience: Jazz and music therapy as modern "rites de passage." In C. Kenny (Ed.), *Listening, playing, creating: Essays on the power of sound.* Albany, NY: State University of New York Press.

Ryff, C. (1989). Happiness is everything or is it? Explorations on the meaning of psychological well-being. *Journal of Personality and Social Psychology, 57*(6), 1069–1081.

Sacks, O. (1995). *An anthropologist on Mars.* New York, NY: Alfred A. Knopf.

Salas, J. (1990). Aesthetic experience in music therapy. *Music Therapy, 9* (1), 1–15.

Schieby, B. (1991). Mia's fourteenth—the symphony of fate: Psychodynamic improvisation therapy with a music therapy student in training. In K. Bruscia (Ed.), *Case studies in music therapy* (pp. 271–290). Pheonixville, PA: Barcelona Publishing.

Schreibman, L., Dawson, G., Stahmer, A., Landa, R., Rogers, S., McGee, G., et al. (2015). Naturalistic developmental behavioral interventions: Empirically validated treatments for Autism Spectrum Disorder. *Journal of Autism and Developmental Disorders, 45*(8), 2411–2428

Schrödinger, E. (1967). *What is life?: With mind and matter and autobiographical sketches.* London, UK: Cambridge University Press. pp. 134–135.

Seligman, M., & Csikszentmihalyi, M. (2000). Positive psychology: An introduction. *American Psychologist, 55*(1), 5–14.

Seligman, M. E. P. (2002). *Authentic happiness: Using the new positive psychology to realize your potential for lasting fulfillment.* New York, NY: Free Press.

Shakespeare, W. (2001). *Hamlet.* The tragical history of Hamlet Prince of Denmark; Act 1, scene 5. New York, NY: Penguin Random House.

Small, C. (1998). *Musicing.* Hanover, NH: Wesleyan University Press.

Smith, D. (2007). *Muses, madmen, and prophets: Rethinking the history, science, and meaning of auditory hallucination.* New York, NY: Penguin Press.

Soshensky, R. (2001). Music therapy and addiction. *Music Therapy Perspectives, 19*(1), pp. 45–52.

Soshensky, R. (2005). Developing a guitar-based approach in Nordoff-Robbins music therapy. *Music Therapy Perspectives, 23*(2), pp. 111–117.

Soshensky, R. (2007). Music therapy for clients with substance use disorders. In B. Crowe & C. Colwell, *Music therapy for children, adolescents and adults with mental disorders.* Silver Spring, MD: American Music Therapy Association pp. 206–223.

Soshensky, R. (2011). Everybody is a star: Performing, recording and community music therapy. *Music Therapy Perspectives, 29*(1), pp. 23–30.

Stige, B. (2002). *Culture-centered music therapy.* Gilsum, NH: Barcelona Publishers.

Stige, B. (2003). *Elaborations toward a notion of community music therapy.* (Doctoral dissertation). Department of Music and Theatre, University of Oslo.

Stokowski, L. (1967, May 11). Addressing an audience at Carnegie Hall, as quoted in the *New York Times.*

Stone, D. (2008). Wounded healing: Exploring the circle of compassion in the helping relationship. *The humanistic psychologist, 36* (1), 45–51.

Storey, D. (n.d.). David Bohm, implicate order and holomovement. Retrieved from https://www.scienceandnonduality.com/david-bohm-implicate-order-and-holomovement/.

Stravinsky, I. (1961). In *The Observer,* October 8, 1961.

Szwed, J. (2012). *So what: The life of Miles Davis.* New York, NY: Random House.

Thayer, A. W., Deiters, H., & Riemann, H. (1928). *The life of Ludwig Van Beethoven (Vol. 3).* Cambridge, UK: Cambridge University Press.

Thomas, J. (1975). *Chasin the Trane: The music and mystique of John Coltrane.* Garden City, NY: Doubleday.

Thoreau, H. D. (2016). *Walden or, life in the woods.* Ballingslöv, Sweden: Wisehouse Classics.

Tolle, E. (2004). *The power of now: A guide to spiritual enlightenment.* Novato, CA: New World Library.

Tramo, M. (2001). Biology of music: Music of the hemispheres. *Science Magazine, 29*(5510), 1920.

Truscott, A. (2015). Experiment confirms quantum theory weirdness. Retrieved from https://phys.org/news/2015-05-quantum-theory-weirdness.html.

Turry, A. (1998). Transference and countertransference in Nordoff-Robbins music therapy. In K. Bruscia (Ed.), *The dynamics of music psychotherapy*, (pp. 181–212). Gisum, NH: Barcelona.

Turry, A. (2001). Supervision in the Nordoff-Robbins training program. In M. Forinash (Ed.), *Music therapy supervision* (pp. 351–378). Gilsum, NH: Barcelona.

Turry, A., & Marcus, D. (2003). Using the Nordoff-Robbins approach to music therapy with adults diagnosed with autism. In D. J. Wiener & L. K. Oxford (Eds.), *Action therapy with families and groups: Using creative arts improvisation in clinical practice*, (pp. 197–228). Washington, DC: APA Books.

Turry, A. (2004). *Music psychotherapy and community music therapy: Questions and considerations*. Unpublished manuscript.

Turry, A. (2005). Music Psychotherapy and Community Music Therapy: Questions and Considerations. *Voices: A World Forum for Music Therapy, 5*(1). https://doi.org/10.15845/voices.v5i1.208

Turry, A. (2016). *What can music do? Rethinking autism through music therapy*. https://www.nyu.edu/about/news-publications/news/2016/july/autism-and-neurodiversity-at-nordoff-robbins-center-for-music-th.html.

Ulanov, A. B. (2005). *Spirit in Jung*. Einsiedeln, Switzerland: Daimon.

Vriend, J., & Dyer, W. (1976). Creatively labeling behavior in individual and group counseling. *Journal of Marital and Family Therapy*, 2(1). https://doi.org/10.1111/j.1752-0606.1976.tb00393.x.

Wagner, F. (1999). *What every music therapist needs to know: How to improvise using the modes and the pentatonics*. https://www.frankdwagner.com/merch. New York, NY: Self-Published manuscript.

Walia, A. (2016). Physicists say consciousness should be considered a state of matter: The "non physical" is real. *Collective evolution*. Retrieved from: https://www.collective-evolution.com/2016/10/28/physicists-say-consciousness-should-be-considered-a-state-of-matter-the-non-physical-is-real/.

Wallis, C. (2005, January 9). The new science of happiness. *Time*.

Weber, R. (1987). Meaning as being in the implicate order philosophy of David Bohm: A conversation. In Basil J. Hiley & D. Peat (Eds.), *Quantum implications: Essays in honour of David Bohm*, pp. 336–350. London: Methuen.

Weir, W. (1999). *In the spirit: Conversations with the spirit of Jerry Garcia*. New York, NY: Three Rivers Press.

Weisman, A. (1995). *Gaviotas: A villiage to reinvent the world*. White River Junction, VT: Chelsea Green Publishing.

Welter, F., & Schonle, P. (1997). *Neurological rehabilitation*. Stuttgart, Germany: Fisher Verlag.

Wheeler, J. A. (1978). "The 'Past' and the 'Delayed-Choice Double-Slit Experiment.'" In A. R. Marlow (Ed.), *Mathematical Foundations of Quantum Theory*. New York, NY: Academic Press. pp. 9–48.

Wigram, T., & Baker, F. (2005). *Songwriting: Methods, techniques and clinical applications for music therapy clinicians, educators and students*. London, UK: Jessica Kingsley Publishers.

Wilber, K. (1985). *No boundary: Eastern and western approaches to personal growth*. Boston, MA, and London: Shambala.

Winnicott, D. W. (1949). Hate in the counter-transference. *The journal of psychotherapy practice and research, 3*(4), 348–356.

Winnecott, D. W. (1966). The location of the cultural experience. *International Journal of Psychoanalysis, 48*, 366–372.

World Health Organization. (2017). Responding to children and adolescents who have been sexually abused. Retrieved from http://www.who.int/reproductivehealth/topics/violence/clinical-response-csa/en/.

Wyatt, W. (2014). *The alchemy of dreams, Volume Two: The universal laws governing dreaming, consciousness and relationships.* Minneapolis, MN: Mill City Press.

Yalom, I. (1995). *The theory and practice of group psychotherapy.* New York, NY: Basic Books.

Yalom, I. (2009). *Gift of therapy: An open letter to a new generation of therapists and their patients.* New York, NY: HarperCollins Publishers.

Yeats, W. B. (1946). *Letters to his son W. B. Yeats and others.* New York, NY: E. P. Dutton and Co.

Zappa, F. (n.d.). theysaidso.com. Retrieved October 8, 2018, from https://theysaidso.com/quote/frank-zappa-music-is-always-a-commentary-on-society.

Zharinova-Sanderson, O. (2005). Promoting integration and socio-cultural change. In M. Pavlicevic & G. Ansdell (Eds.), *Community music therapy*, pp. 233–248. London: Jessica Kingsley Publishers.

Zollo, P. (2012). Bob Dylan: The Paul Zollo interview. *American songwriter.* Retrieved from http://americansongwriter.com/2012/01/bob-dylan-the-paul-zollo-interview-3/.

Zuckerkandl, Viktor. (1973). *Sound and symbol. Vol. 2: Man the musician.* Princeton, NJ: Princeton University Press.

Index

About the Author

Rick Soshensky, MA, LCAT, MT-BC, NRMT, is a nationally known music therapist. He has published numerous journal articles and textbook chapters and has lectured both nationally and internationally. He operates Hudson Valley Creative Arts Therapy Studio (www.HVCATS.org), a Music Therapy Studio in his hometown of Kingston, New York, and teaches in the music therapy departments at SUNY New Paltz and Molloy College. His work has been featured in the *New York Times*, on National Public Radio, Fox Radio, and numerous other print, TV, radio, and web media.

Rick has lived his entire life in the world of music, performed for the Queen of England, and played gigs with Ella Fitzgerald and the Four Tops. As part of the New York City music scene in the eighties and early nineties, Rick wrote songs, recorded, and performed in venues throughout the country. In the mid-nineties, Rick shifted direction, enrolled in New York University to complete his master's degree in music therapy, and began applying his musical talents for the growth and healing of his clients.